Cancer, my BFF:)!

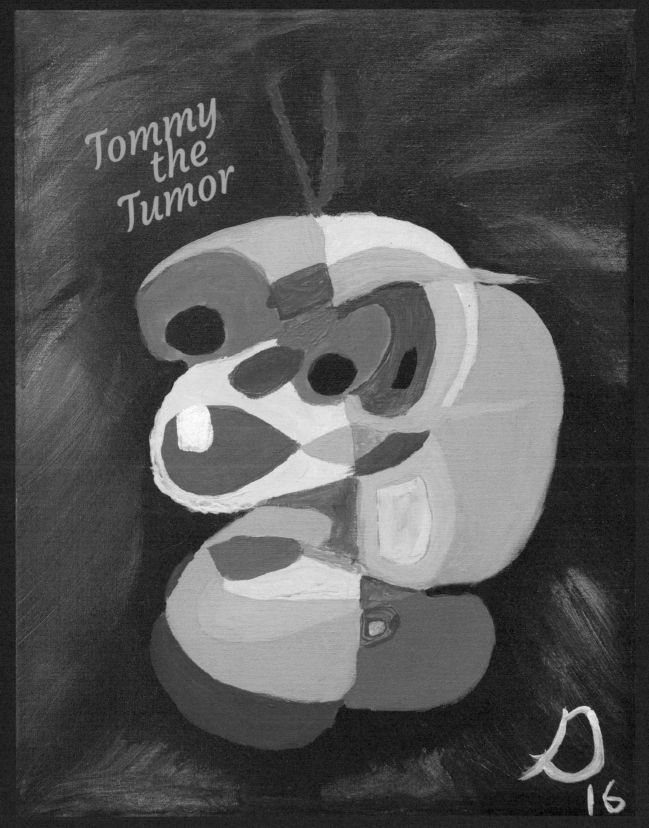

Tommy the Tumor

Dennis G. Whittaker

Archway Publishing books may be ordered through booksellers or by contacting:

Archway Publishing
1663 Liberty Drive
Bloomington, IN 47403
www.archwaypublishing.com
1 (888) 242-5904

Because of the dynamic nature of the Internet, any web addresses or links contained in this book may have changed since publication and may no longer be valid. The views expressed in this work are solely those of the author and do not necessarily reflect the views of the publisher, and the publisher hereby disclaims any responsibility for them.

Any people depicted in stock imagery provided by Getty Images are models, and such images are being used for illustrative purposes only.
Certain stock imagery © Getty Images.

Project Editor: Donna J. Steen
Production Editor:
Copy editor:
Photographer: Dennis G. Whittaker
Cover Design: Donna J. Steen
Artwork Design: Donna J. Steen
Page Layout: Dennis G. Whittaker
            Donna J. Steen

ISBN: 978-1-4808-8561-5 (sc)
ISBN: 978-1-4808-8562-2 (hc)
ISBN: 978-1-4808-8563-9 (e)

Library of Congress Control Number: 2019920095

Print information available on the last page.

Archway Publishing rev. date: 01/30/2020

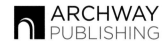

Table of Contents

Introduction

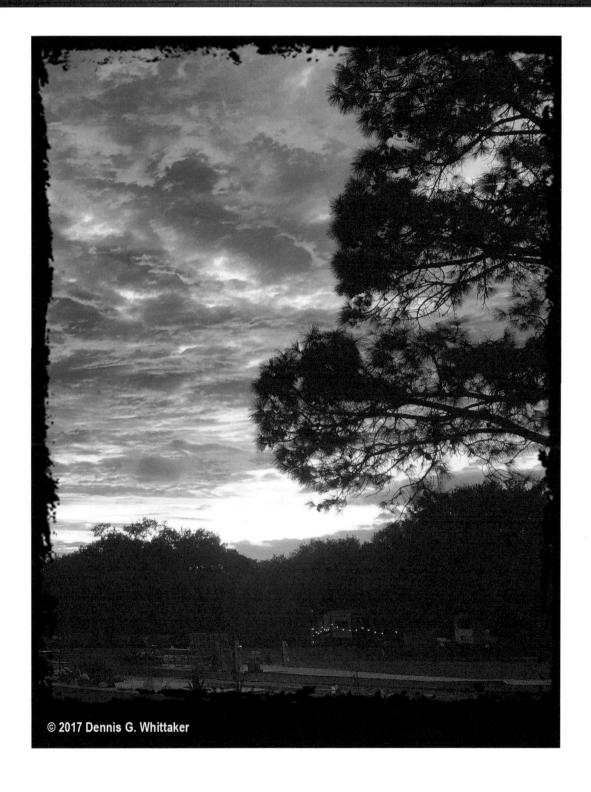

© 2017 Dennis G. Whittaker

Forever an optimist, Dennis Whittaker has always managed to persevere through all of life's challenges, surviving everything, including the truths, treatments and recovery from stage 4 cancer.

His mind over matter approach shines through all the ups and downs of this harrowing ordeal with his honest and humorous insights into the realities of this dreaded disease and related artifacts (aka: side effects.)

About the book:

Cancer, my BFF, is a refreshing insight into the realities of surviving and accepting any of the major and debilitating nuisances presented during our lives.

This book explores many of the hidden truths and realities of each stage of the entire process of treatment, recovery of the body, and what may be the toughest part, recovery of the mind, spirit and our little friend Mr. or Mrs. Ego.

The title says it all, as Dennis accepted every reality on his journey with a keen desire to make cancer his truly best friend forever.

Intertwined with "Before and After" tales, some hand spun "Quipets" and his personal photographs, the story will provide an honest and humorous look into how to make the best of any of life's funky turns.

"Gotta Breathe! May as well Enjoy it:)!"

dgw

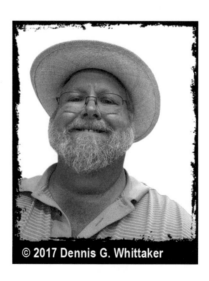

© 2017 Dennis G. Whittaker

The Pre-Forward

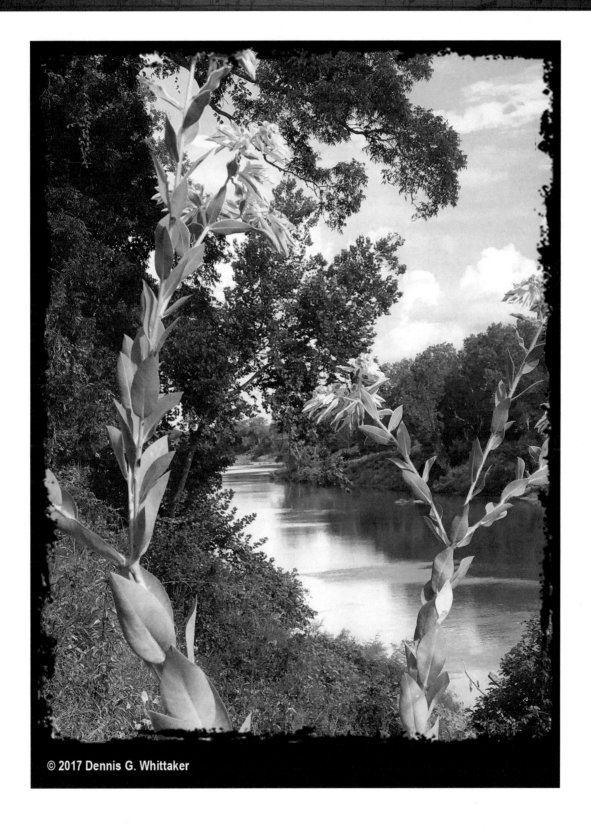

© 2017 Dennis G. Whittaker

Well, like it or not, it is 2017 as we speak. So, what does that mean exactly? Heck if I know.

What I do know is that things aren't as they used to be. The reference for things one is not allowed to speak on the telly has been replaced with a new list of vulgarities. Ones that are more vulgar are now on the telly on a regular basis. Even our politicians are using the F-Word to agree or, more often, disagree amongst themselves.

This of course, puts somebody like me in a funny spot. It would be much simpler to write my story if I didn't have a care in the world as to who I might upset or offend. Heck, that may help me sell some books.

On the other hand, this book is intended to be a number of things, but IT IS NOT intended to be insulting, upsetting, infuriating, aggravating, exasperating, shocking, irritating, demeaning or any other feeling that affects one's blood pressure in a negative way.

On the other, other hand, it is intended to be real, honest, aloof and humorous, and hopefully inspirational in its own way. That is why I have rated it as HH for Honest & Humorous!

Through the advice of a dear friend, I decided that the best way to bridge the gaps as an author in 2017, is to reference these potentially offensive words in the appropriate context, thus ensuring the story's integrity. However, to avoid over use and potential abuse of these words, they will be shortened to an acronym, which you as the reader can manipulate to your hearts content.

Forward

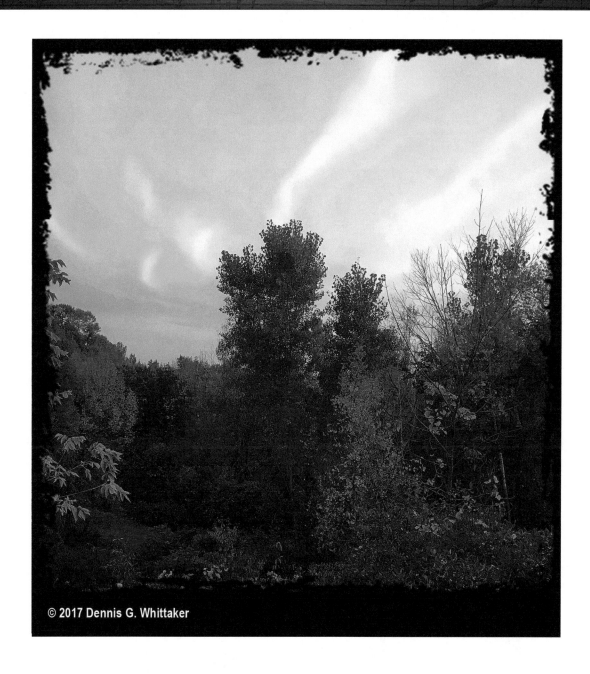

© 2017 Dennis G. Whittaker

Life, as always, is moving along at over 1000 miles an hour. The vicious circle of earn, spend, earn more, spend more continues to spiral out of control, to the point that we work to live instead of the other way around.

I believe this lifestyle to be more common than we care to admit. It is my hope, amongst other things, to provide a new perspective to this cycle of life.

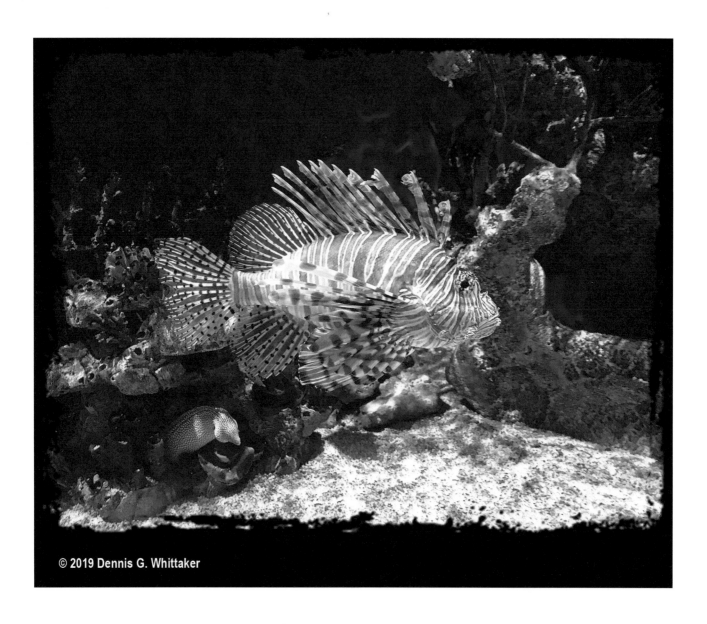

© 2019 Dennis G. Whittaker

If this sounds familiar to you, then please read on and see why my fight with Stage 4 Squamous Cell Cancer At Base Of Tongue[Q2] became my best friend.

I know, I know. What can possibly be good about being close to death, tied to a host of medical professionals, IV's, radical radiation and losing what in my case was the most important part of my brain function, to something called a "Major Neurocognitive Disorder" which impacts my memory, attention, ability to complete many tasks, and has basically castrated me from all of the incredibly fascinating and productive problem solving that made me such a valued asset in my brain.

For the historians, today is November 17th, 2017.

My cancer has been in remission for almost a year, which is totally freaking awesome, and why I can now share some stories with you, and why I thank my new BFF for giving me a new chance to regroup, re-think (that may be overstated) and create a new life.

Yeah, I know that you know that this story will be a bittersweet one. It has taken everything I could muster since my diagnosis to find the silver lining in my cancer cloud. The biggest challenge has been to simply accept who and what I am.

While being no better than my fellow Homo sapiens, I was a legend in my own mind. So, losing what in my case was the most important part of my brain function was and still is devastating. This impacts my memory, attention, ability to complete many tasks, and has displaced me from the incredibly fascinating and productive skills I had been recognized for and that had previously defined myself, well, to myself????

I could solve most any business dilemma or manufacturing challenge. I was a good spouse and father, but not a great one most of the time. After all, my workaholic tendencies and living in my brain made family and friends a second choice to allow for the true love of my life, which was my brain.

So, let's just say that I have had a bit of a falling out with my old self. I simply can't count on the creative brain trust that bridged both sides of my mind into an amazing CPU. My ability to make a living has changed dramatically and I don't expect to make 6 figures again until a loaf of bread is $22 as is a jug of milk or pound of cheese.

So, let me share my story that bridges where I came from to where I have been and ultimately how I landed in the best and happiest place and time I have ever known. I will share the best and worst of my life and my experiences, not that they are better or more important than anyone else's, but maybe it can shed some light on some ways to deal with your own.

B1　Dennis, the Navigator — Before . . .

I usually did most of the driving when I was in the car. My destinations and maps were printed and ready to go, and my sense of direction was keen. I was rarely lost, hence I was rarely late.

Driving a car is a simple thing to do.

Dennis, the Navigator — After . . .

I no longer drive. To this, I sincerely extend a warm "You're Welcome' to anyone that has been on the same roads as I, while my wife moves us along, safe and steady at about 60ish mph.

The only real driving risk now, outside of everybody else on the road, is if / when I help.

I like to help, it is a part of my soul, or at least it was.

Now, it is a pain in the butt. Driving a motor vehicle requires 100% of a normal human brain's ability to properly and safely manage.

This statement is supported by the ugly statistics that fall under "DUI" or "Driving under the Influence," "TWD" or Texting While Driving, "SWD" or Sleeping While Driving, and "YATKWD" or Yelling at the Kids While Driving.

As is well understood at this point, I no longer have access to 100% of my brain's abilities, which has led to a new thing called "BADWD" or Being Around Dennis While Driving.

I am not sure which statute in the law books of any State in the southwest clearly states the harm that can and will come from BADWD or the related fines and prison terms, but I can say that this is just as serious as any other safety related concerns governed in the Southwest. To be clear, when BADWD is in play, the following will happen eventually, or, more likely, all the freakin' time:

Sudden panic to take this turn at all costs!

A very long and arduous detour because of this sudden panic:(

An angry person screaming, "I DON'T KNOW!" Which of course is me.

A different angry person screaming "YOU IDIOT" (etc., etc., etc., etc., etc.,) Which of course is the person driving for an extra hour due to the wrong turn in or around Albuquerque.

Post-Forward

The Final Chapter (Kinda?) — Why Cancer is My BFF!

"Day's Are Numbers" *by The Alan Parsons Project*

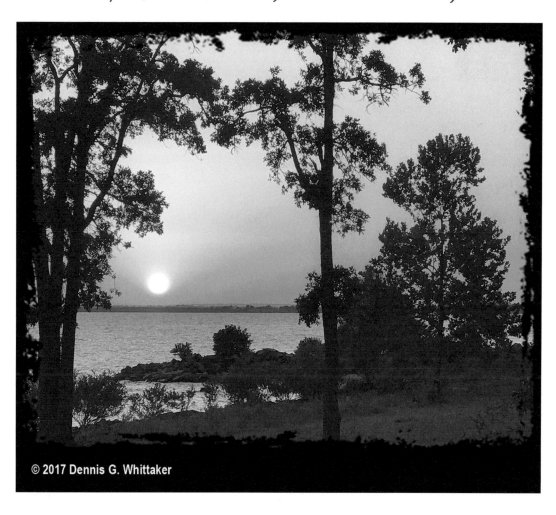

© 2017 Dennis G. Whittaker

Yeah, I know it is kinda odd to present the end of the story first, but I have what my wife and I lovingly refer to as "AssHoleBergers Syndrome"- AHB. Going Forward (no offense to anyone please,) this apparently gives me some kind of birthright to not fit into to what everybody else considers to be normal, so why start now, right?

Asperger's Syndrome Manifestations:

After being married for about 27 years, my wife decided to research and find out why I was so standoffish, didn't allow anything in life to really get to me, including the death of loved ones, and why I seemed to rarely listen to what she was saying. Hence the Reference to "AssHoleBergers" (AHB going forward) Syndrome.

Do Artifacts Exist?

Interestingly, after cancer treatments were completed and I was Cancer Free (Yeah!) I went through some crazy depression, anxiety and an entire host of what I lovingly refer to as "The Artifacts (Please see "The Artifacts – AKA – The Side Effects" chapter for more details.) My Psychiatrist immediately diagnosed me with that exact thing and said the treatment plan is the same for my new problems as for the "AHB" Thing.

How Nice and Convenient.

Maybe you landed on this book because you or a loved one has or had cancer or maybe was just diagnosed with it. You are full of apprehension, questions, concerns, possibly some anger, bitterness or resentment. Trust me, if you haven't already done so you will go through all 12 stages of some yet to be identified Cancer Feeling / Thought Process starting the moment the Doctor looks inside and sees a cancerous tumor instead of what he expected to see. My cancer was a squamous cell tumor at the base of my tongue.

So, let's get back to the end of the story. You can read all about my journey through the jungle after you get to enjoy the punch line.

Here Is What You Need To Know:

Cancer will change your life – Some of us will die in the process (Damn Cancer!), others, in increasing numbers, will survive, and for some of us, our quality of life will be so much better than ever before, even with these "Artifacts" that can drastically change your day to day. For me, I became disabled, just not the kind that requires a wheelchair or to be hooked up to an IV every week.

Mine is more from what they call Chemo Brain, which, in my case is the same diagnosis folks get from traumatic brain injuries like concussions. For me, it feels like there is a black hole in my brain. If I try to add 37 + 44, after adding the 4 and 7 to get 11, go to carry the one, and I have no clue what the first digits were. I am now in need of one of those calculator thingies.

I used to sit in executive meetings and listen to folks build a scenario through multiple stages and 5 minutes later I would tell them the answer. They banged on their calculators for a couple minutes and came up with the same answer. After a couple of episodes, they gave up and trusted me.

So, the math side of my brain has gone AWOL, my social skills and desires went on the same holiday, and now "Mr. Teflon™" has some anger management issues.

At 55 years old when I was diagnosed, I was very much a workaholic. 70-hour weeks were the norm. With a high school diploma, I was able to make 6 figures most of my life, owned businesses, was a VP in a $70M company, and re-invented my career every 3 years starting in high school. I loved my work, did it well, and have an absolute ton of highlights in my career, which may be another book to itself, as this one really isn't about that.

Obviously, the cancer did a bit of a number on me, so to speak.

So, what do we do when life gives us lemons? We make the most amazing sweet and tangy lemonade. The kind that stops Arizona summers in their tracks. There are a number of sayings that we all have, like "Turn Our Frown Upside Down," "Don't Make a Mountain Out of a Molehill", "Don't Waste Your Time and Money Making Tollhouse Cookies Without Real Creamery Butter" (Why this isn't considered a mortal sin is so confusing, isn't it?) And "Since Fresh Cheese Curds Are the Single Best Food On Planet Earth, Why Aren't They Available in Every Store on The Planet?!"

In other words, let's regroup and be willing to really explore our priorities.

For me, I spent my entire life chasing the next audition, the next bonus, the next sale, the next life changing business solution. I made a lot of money, and unfortunately managed to lose it all. No excuses.

Here We Go!

- We sold pretty much everything that we owned
- We rented out our house
- We purchased a 20' travel trailer to call our home
- We traded in two cars on a Nissan Pathfinder to pull our trailer
- We built a fun life bouncing around from campground to campground
- We buy farm fresh eggs when we can find them
- We get farm fresh fruits and pick our own berries when we can
- We sleep better
- We get a kick out of feeding deer where it is allowed, taking time to photograph our experiences as we go
- We cook almost all of our meals at home, eating out as we drive from place to place
- We eat only whole foods, sprouted nuts and grains, chicken without Carrageenan or Citrus Flour, and the most amazing homemade breads, toaster muffins and blueberry pancakes (Yes, my wife makes all this in our 20' trailer!)
- We spend quality time with our friends and family. As a workaholic, these things were always a distraction to what I was working on. Not so any more. These people are really amazing.

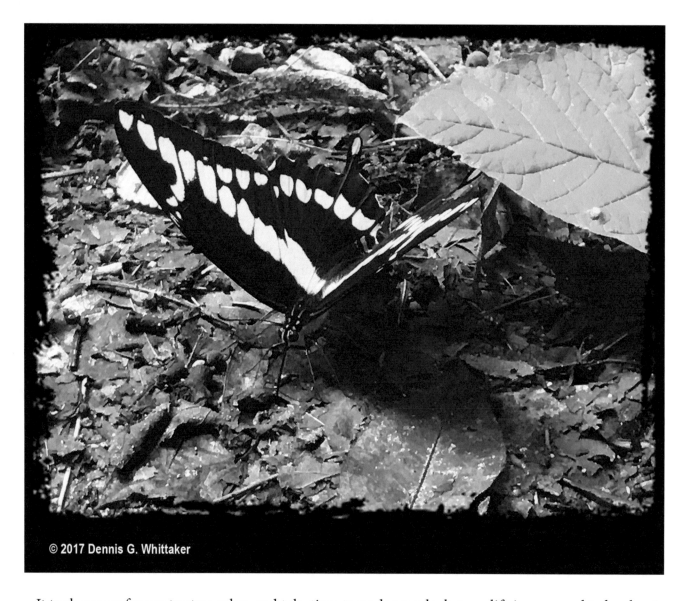

It took cancer for me to stop, relax, and take time to understand what my life is supposed to be about. I have lived in a million-dollar house and drove a Benz and I now live in an $18K trailer and drive a Nissan®. Life has never been better. If I chose this lifestyle 10 years ago, I could have paid cash for all of this and worked on the road. Seeing the sights, breathing the air, and yeah, sorry, stop to smell the roses, the forests, the skunks (it happens) and all the sweet scents that life has to offer.

My wife and I are closer (not just because of our tiny trailer) than we ever have been, I am starting to build the kind of relationships with my kids that they deserved the past 30 years, and love landing in the hometown of our family and friends. We stay in some of the most beautiful places in a Thousand Trails or Encore Campground, our National Parks, Corp Of Engineer Parks, National Forests and State Parks. I even called my mother-in-law "mom" for the first time in 32 years. She says I am a billion times better than I used to be.

It is good to live outside of my head more often, as it was a pretty lonely place to be.

We live a simple life, we stay on budget, we take care of our stuff and I feel more proud of my accomplishments than when I helped build businesses with the unique business solutions only us "AHB" Folks can dream up.

So, what if I can't dream up and create custom software, customer service models that drove a business to be one of the best on the planet, and provided insight found only in the funny perspective and angles that were uniquely mine anymore? What good is a life that is moving so fast all day every day, and where kids and grandkids birthdays are an obligation (can we go now?)

While I certainly wouldn't wish cancer on anyone, 'cause trust me, it is a harrowing ordeal, I do strongly suggest that you take time right now to stop, relax and discover what your true priorities are! Make some adjustments, save some money and make sure that every breath you take will fill you with the fun, fascination and love that comes when you follow your dreams instead of your 5-year plan that include a big house, a TV in every room including the water closet, and a car that can go 165 MPH when the max speed limit is 75. (Heck, even my smart car could go 75 mph on the highway)

There is a lot more to this story, so grab your favorite drink, put on some comfy clothes, and settle into your favorite place to read. I hope that you will find this tale to be both honest and humorous. If so, please share the experience with your circle of friends and family. If not, please file your concerns to the following non-existent email address:

DennisWhittakerIsntVeryFunnyAtAll@nodomainwhatsoever.com

Mr. Teflon™ here, with today's quick tips on how to use your AHB and empathy to good use. Please be careful, as this must be used with skill and honest intentions. Otherwise you're just gonna piss people off all the time. I know this from personal experience. So let's talk about empathy. Pre-Cancer, empathy was this amazing business tool that I was gifted with. It was like my second weapon in my one – two punch. It worked like this. The customer, associate, driver, etc., was enraged, upset and screaming. This demonstration meant absolutely nothing to me. If anything, and from time to time, it was somewhat entertaining. I had to keep myself from pointing and laughing at these people. However, I did care about what caused them to temporarily lose their sanity.

This was like food for me. If the entertainment was pretty good, and the cause was a challenge, I would likely jump in and find a solution. Not because I wanted the show to stop, but because there is a lot of rewarding things I can do with the money when I fix a problem this person had, and maybe every customer had. It really comes in handy when you don't become part of the problem, which is usually what happens when the entertainer gets personal and starts telling you what an amazingly stupid person you turned out to be.

Calling Mr. Teflon™, please pick up the white paging phone for an important message! Mr. Teflon™, are you there?

Nope, he has been replaced by,,,,,,,,,,wait for it,,,,,,, Mr. Basket Case!

This froody new dude is a lot of things, just not Mr. Teflon™. If videotaped in slow motion he would look like a helium balloon that was filled with helium, then released without tying it off.

In other words, I am now all over the place emotionally.

So, let's talk about empathy Post-Cancer, shall we?

I now have an entirely new library of feelings and emotions. These new-found things range from "That was pretty cool!" To "That was very interesting" to "WTF!!!!!"

Empathy was such a cool tool before, and now it takes on a whole new life. I understand and feel what others are going through. I am still undecided if this is wicked cool or just plain annoying. Now I have this new 3rd dimension to my daily life.

I used to be the king of managing the Catch 22 Scenarios, which are those nasty scenarios where it always seems that you're screwed no matter which way you decide to go.

Having no empathy, there were NO WRONG DECISIONS! Not exactly true, but my AHB kept me out of that place where you could find me talking to myself, kinda like this; "You idiot, why didn't you do it the other way. I told you to go the other way, and you just wouldn't listen. I hate you right now! Now what am I gonna do??"

Chapter 1

"The Sound of Silence" *by Simon & Garfunkel, and Disturbed*

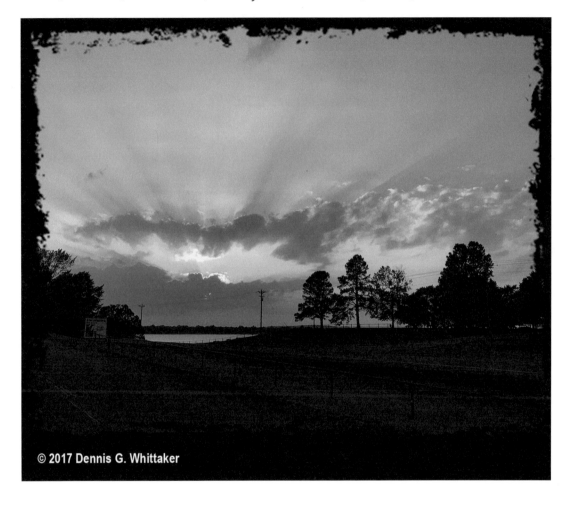

© 2017 Dennis G. Whittaker

I have always been gifted at seeing the very best in life. While life is so much better today, it doesn't mean that I didn't like and enjoy my life prior. I was somewhat of a madman Pre-Cancer. It was so important to me to be the most knowledgeable person in the room, and often (not always, as I have had the honor to work with some incredibly gifted people throughout my life) enjoyed giving myself credit for being the smartest person in the room.

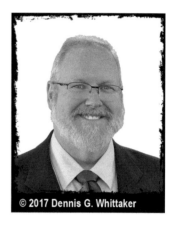

I could visualize any process or business dilemma, immediately see its shortcomings and provide a solution on the spot. When the stakeholders were in agreement, I would build the process and any related supporting elements like slogans, logos, spreadsheets, marketing and training. The solution would be all wrapped with a bow and delivered for review often by the next day.

One of my many roles was to be the company clown, not that I was amusing so much, but I was the master juggler. I always had numerous projects in play at any time, and rarely did one of them miss a beat. It was common for me to have well over 10 fairly major projects rolling at the same time.

In my old life, and once upon a time, my employees referred to me as "Mr. Teflon™." Once again, AHB was on my side.

Two Examples:

1. We had a large industrial oven to cure paints and inks on various products. The control had several programs for the various profiles needed to properly cure something. One day, an employee, in tears, came to me to let me know that he had selected the wrong profile, and all of the customers plastic products are ruined. Funny thing about plastic and heat, right? He fully expected to be fired on the spot for causing a $5K dollar mistake. Instead, we calmly walked over to review the situation, and I asked the employee to think about what he thought we could do to ensure that a mistake like this would never happen again. In other words, it's not your fault for making a mistake! Obviously, we have a process problem that needs to be resolved. The next morning the employee came to me with a smile, and a piece of paper with his idea. Two hours later we had a hinged reminder that was mounted to the controller that simply stated, "Please Verify Profile Prior To Starting This Oven." I thanked him warmly and told him that his idea would likely save us tens of thousands of dollars in the future and gave him a high five!

2. There was a mezzanine above the front offices in my building. It was full of industrial shelving I picked up at an auction. As it didn't come with instructions, or the required braces, the entire floor of shelves fell like dominoes. 4 rows, 20' long. It sounded like a plane had crashed into our building. Loud enough that our ears were still ringing 15 minutes later. Everyone was freaking out, trying to figure out what happened and what we should do. I calmly stood up, walked to the mezzanine door (greeted with a nice gust of dusty wind) and walked up the stairs to see what happened. No big deal, we had a problem which provided us with a learning opportunity to grow from. Life is always providing such wonderful lessons.

As these things go, the logic and mathematical sparks I used to have, (the ones that went AWOL) weren't the only things that changed so dramatically after cancer.

I ended up with a new personality, mind set and list of priorities. After working like a madman for decades and ending up in about the same place financially as when I was 25, it occurred to me that maybe there were more important things to focus on than feeding my brain and my ego. Again, I made lots of money over the years, but managed to lose it all, no excuses.

Today I focus on living. My wife has someone to talk to and to share her life with. My dog Hado and I are now best buds, when in the past he was just a big expensive possession. I take time to visit with my sisters and kids, both on the phone and in person. We live frugally and happily in a small travel trailer. Small enough that every time we buy something new, we need to discard something to manage our space and weight.

While the results are very rewarding, they came at a high cost to my ego and did a number on my emotions. It took a very long time to adapt to the new me, and to accept that I may never again produce the world class solutions that have had a significant impact on the industries that I served. After all, I do remember the rush that comes from creating something of value with the only raw materials being those stored in my brain!

It took four or five different anti-depressants and other drug cocktails to treat my depression which isn't gone, it is just much better. Sounds like I will be on Prozac for the rest of my days.

Mr. Teflon™ still makes appearances now and then, but mostly he keeps to himself. My base personality is shifted. I am much more likely to yell at someone for being inconsiderate or doing something that isn't in the spirit of things. Anger is pretty much a new emotion for me, and while, at times it feels good to express it, my wife is happy to remind me that I may incite some road rage, or for someone to slice a tire or two.

I love projects. The more the merrier. For me, projects were my way to express and impress. I could look at pretty much anything and see with crystal clarity, how it could be improved upon.

I would tear the problem apart like a Lego® kit with pieces, analyze it, melt it all down and put it together with the 6 pieces that actually make it work best.

I did this with manufacturing processes, equipment design, software solutions and any business or customer service process.

It was easier for me to do the "Steve Jobs" with many of these projects. No point in asking what people needed, as they don't know they need something that they have never seen or comprehended previously.

I love hating projects, if that makes any sense.

I am cursed with still having the ability to see a better solution to a problem.

It is exciting to see the formation of a new project, until I spend 10 or 20 or 40 or more hours trying to bring it to life. I am now trying to figure out how to build that 873-piece LEGO® kit, but I am now colorblind as I have no use of any 3 dimensional concepts. I have neuropathy in both hands so my ability to pick up the parts and put them together is both painful and frustrating.

I start over, and over and over to a point of frustration, anger and hatred that is unmanageable and unimaginable.

I am no longer talking about how to incorporate 10 independent process steps and craft them into a single software process.

These major projects (Pronounced "Insurmountable Hurdles") were the simplest of tasks a couple of years ago.

- Build a step for our trailer. Two steps, 5-6" rise 24" wide and 24" deep. $74 in materials, over 20 different designs. Finally bought the wood and a saw and built them without the help of any real design
- Mount the various charging devices, antennas, etc. under our table top = Catastrophic failure. Looking to find the nerve to start over.
- Mount a waste tank to the back of the trailer
- Build simple shelves in our closets

Every one of these simple projects have overtaken my every thought for days at a time. They have each taken multiple designs, a high cost ($) to redo and redo again prior to having an acceptable solution.

Chapter 2

Dennis, The Party Animal ?????

"Mary Had a Little Lamb", *Traditional*

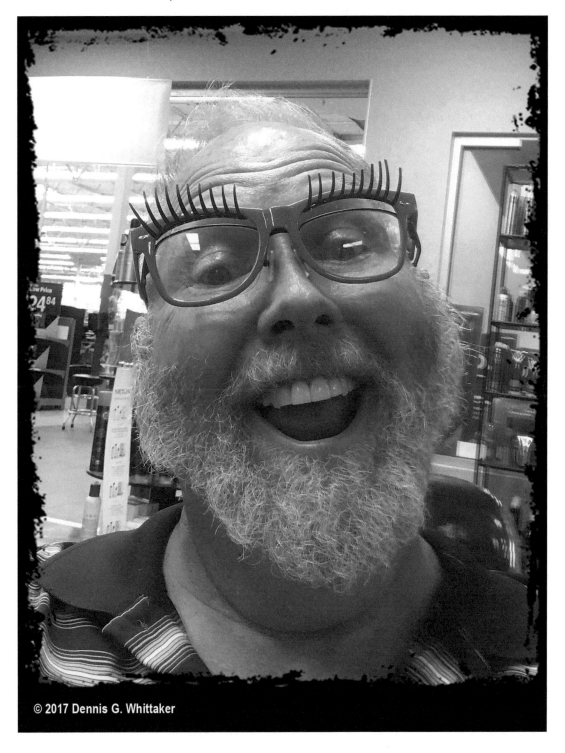

© 2017 Dennis G. Whittaker

For the mathematicians, today is Saturday, November 25th, which is two days after Thanksgiving. This is one math problem I can still solve without a calculator. This fills me with a calming warmth, as it proves that I am still good for something technical in nature:)

Ahhh. Warm and relaxed, coffee in hand, this should be a good time to tell you about my previous success as a party animal.

This is also a tale about my "Social Split Personality Disorder." I am fully aware of the main characters, both of them.

Everyone that has ever seen the movie knows this about that:

> Anyone with more than one personality and less than three will always have a timid (lamb) personality married to an outgoing, often borderline aggressive (lion) personality.

They tend to get along pretty well with a handful of exceptions that people always categorize as "passive / aggressive," which is a title we earned from time to time over the years:)

A Lamb's Tale:

Everybody I have ever met in a social situation, at least those that weren't centered around my work, knows, without question, that I have AHB.

This is not to say that they are all experts or even peripherally aware of Aspergers.

What they do know, is the minute that I am in a purely social situation amongst strangers, I will be the person that stands out as the person in the room that doesn't stand out at all, which in a funny sort a way, makes me stand out like a sore thumb.

Making small talk is painful for me, which is pronounced "Awkward!!" When I do say something, the reactions fully support that I am completely out of line, out of place, and out of time. Speaking of which, "Please excuse me, as it is time for me to escape to refill my drink regardless of how empty my glass may or may not be." (Run away!!!!)

With reflection, this aspect of my life has been one of the biggest drains on me. Most folks can't wait for the next party, BBQ, wedding, or pretty much any reason to get together and socialize. I, on the other hand, was always 150% conflicted by this. It was a sick obsession.

The idea of making new friends and being the life of the party was always appealing to me. At 56 this appeal has finally run its course. I am simply too tired to sign up for any more abuse or failure in this department.

My two best friends came to me completely outside of a group get together.

My college friend needed a ride home after we both sold concessions at an ASU (Arizona State University) football game. We enjoyed each other's company and started finding more and more reasons to pal around.

My college friend called me to ask "When are we gonna go to Monti's La Casa Vieja for a steak dinner? Let's go tonight!" It took him about 15 minutes to convince me that the world would not fall apart, if at 18, I told my mom I wouldn't be home for dinner. Turns out he was right:)!

These gentlemen have been riding in the drivers and/or passenger seats of my life back to the late 1970's and are always ready for another journey! I love you guys!

This lamb side of my personality has changed exactly 0%. So, kindly send any party or social invitations to someone that will be less conspicuous at your event, as my social silence may not be acceptable or appreciated.

The Lion's Tale:

I may have mentioned that I was a workaholic. In that life, you may have joined me for some "Truly Exceptional" training or to enjoy one of many worthwhile presentations. If I had the good fortune to have worked with you, you may or may not have immediately thought of AHB.

I regress,

This was my DOMAIN!

I have rehearsed every handshake, every little joke, how and when to really make a point, and have already enjoyed several standing ovations. Well, maybe in my mind at least:)

The point is, my performance was scripted in advance, scheduled, lots of reminders, and perfectly and completely choreographed.

If what I believe is somewhat of a contradiction to my AHB, this was a part of my life that brought me a great deal of joy and success. My business persona was warm, outgoing and friendly. Moreover, I had the confidence of a lion that just loved to roar!

I really can't tell you how I would do today in front of 5-50 strangers with one of my award-winning dances. I expect, at best, I would be a lion's cub, or possibly a freakish mix of a lamb and lion's cub.

My lion's ego is chiming in, something about "Shut Up Dennis! Until you get out there and give it a shot, you will never really know how it will feel to perform again. Who knows, maybe it's like riding a bike? Get out there and roar like your old self!!!!"

Unfortunately, my lion voice is but a whisper these days, as the lamb has taken control of the motivational center. Living up to his "quiet as a lamb" character, it is now so perfectly quiet, it is truly deafening.

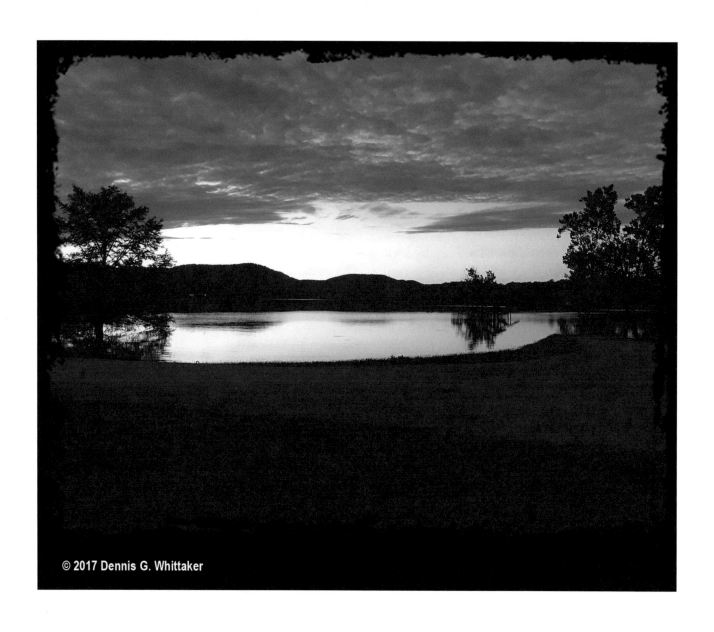

Chapter 3

How Did This Happen to Me & Why?

"Everything Gives You Cancer" *by Joe Jackson*

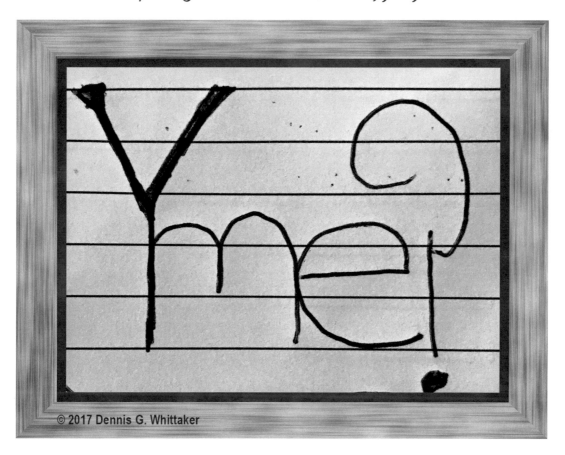

© 2017 Dennis G. Whittaker

You're right! Folks always ask, "Why ME?" When bad things happen, even the simply benign things like picking the wrong line at the store or when you miss a traffic light. And yes, I certainly went through the process when I learned I had cancer.

So, there is simply no point in trying to understand the "Why ME?" question until we have enough empirical (facts, figures, other things we can't argue with) evidence to give us an idea of what may have caused this, spend some honest reflection time, and then start guessing what went wrong and who is responsible. It seems like there is always someone else at the core of our problems, but the truth is it is almost always includes ourselves as a participant.

So with my cancer, it kinda went like this:

1. I felt unhealthy – For me it was a sore throat and being tired all the time. I fell asleep on the couch regularly between 6:30 and 7:30 in the evening.

2. Saw a doctor.

3. Some routine tests were performed and I was laughed out of the office to make room for someone worthy of all the doctor's amazing education. NOTE: Don't leave the office until you get something to go on or find a new doctor. If you're sick you deserve to be properly evaluated and treated before things get out of control as they did with me. I lost 3 months between this visit and being diagnosed with Stage 4 Cancer.

4. I went to my dentist when my breath was so bad that my wife wouldn't stay in the same room with me. It was time to see my friendly dentist to have this foul odor yanked out of my mouth, but there was nothing wrong with my teeth. He suggested I make an appointment with a specialist. Got it, time to do some research.

5. Saw another doctor to discuss the problems and to come to the hypothesis that this was all caused by another and more serious round of Reflux. But let's run a snake down your nose and see what we find. This is the point that this doctor's office turned into a haunted house. When he pulled the snake out, he was pale and looked like he had seen a ghost. He couldn't possibly refer me fast enough or get me out of his office any sooner. It was like my cancer was contagious and he wanted no part of it.

6. Saw a specialist that focuses on cancer and related surgeries. This man was so sincere and warm. His concern was evident from the time we said hi, to the time he sent me up for some pictures of my tumor. He had me scheduled for a biopsy the next morning which proved that I had a squamous cell carcinoma at the base of my tongue. It had a certain marker in it that was tied to HPV (Human Papillomavirus.)

7. Saw another specialist. Well, you can do this after your insurance company spends a few days reviewing all of this so they will approve the costs going forward.

8. Learn for real that you have Stage 4 Cancer. No worries, we can fix this! Once again, I see that I am building a dream team with medical professionals that know their stuff, move quickly and all have a way of making you feel as comfortable as possible as you go through the process.

9. Next day it is time to install a Medi-Port to make it more productive to deliver the Chemo and to take blood. And then the chemo starts the very next day.

Now, there is much more to this story but for now, we have enough to get back to that ugly "Why ME?" thing.

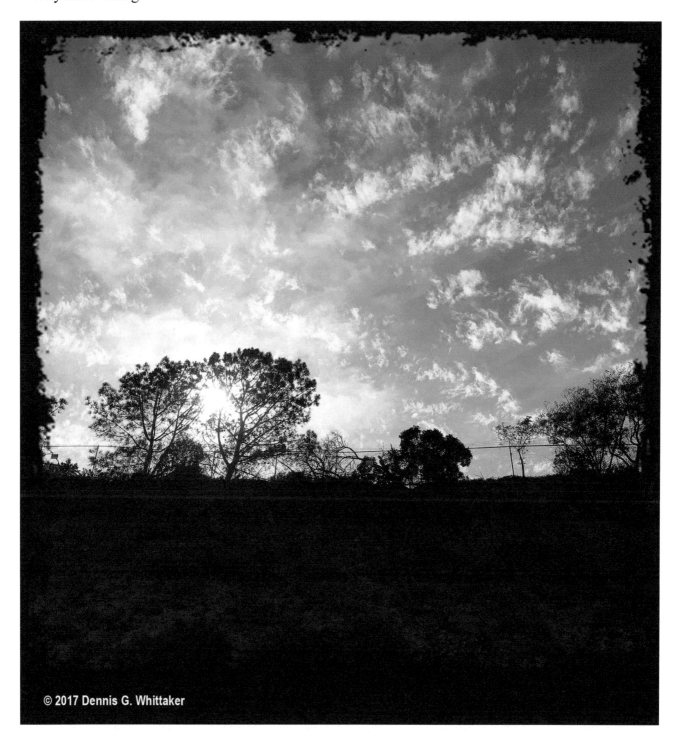

Most folks get this type of cancer by one, two or all three of these contributors:

1. Smoking too much (I have never smoked, save the times in Hong Kong and Shanghai when someone offered me a Cuban cigar to choke on.)

2. Drinking too much (I have never been much of a drinker, save the times the ASU Marching Band went to a bar to rehydrate after the football games)

3. Having contact with another human being through kissing, loving, etc. at any time in your lifetime. You don't even need to take your clothes off to get this form of an STD. In other words, who knows who is to "blame" for this being the cause of my cancer. Most folks process it simply through their system, but good folks like me take it seriously and end up with cancer.

So, "Why ME?" At the end of the day it simply doesn't matter. Knowing who ran the stop sign and dinged your car, who is causing the slow lane at the store, or why somebody ALWAYS wins the big lotto other than me, rarely helps. It certainly can't be used to reshape history or take the physical or emotional pain out of the situation. For me, I accepted my fate and focused on what had to happen to save my cute, not so little butt from an early grave. And make no mistake, you will not be alone on your journey. You will get to know all about how important my wife was as a caregiver and best friend, all the doctors and their staffs that worked tirelessly to help me through the entire process, and of course all my family, friends, and co-workers that stuck by my side through thick and thin. Mostly thick, like a milkshake that you can never ever drink through a straw even after it has melted.

"Ya Gotta Breath, Ya May As Well Enjoy It!"

WHAT IS HPV?

HPV, Human Papillomavirus is considered to be a sexually transmitted disease.

They say that everyone that has ever been physically close to another person, even through a simple kiss, will be exposed to this virus.

Most people ignore this virus, and it simply comes and goes.

Some of us, however, hold onto the virus like a treasured gift or memory.

We carry it around in our body somehow, sometimes for years or even decades.

Boredom eventually sets in for the HPV, and it decides to go forth and multiply, so to speak, in one of many forms of cancer.

The good news part of this little story is that cancers caused by the HPV virus are more treatable than others.   (Yeah!!!)

Warm, Friendly and comfortable in my own shoes. I would happily walk up to just about anybody and start a conversation. At least in a business setting. Can't explain it, but I never knew what to say in a basic social gathering or party. I was the dufus in the corner waiting for someone to talk to me. I often left parties early, making excuses about the kids, the dogs, the laundry, the project, etc.

On any given day, I could approach 30 – 50 folks, see how they were doing, start a conversation about anything I could pick up from them. I didn't care about the topic, if I had a link of any kind I was all in! "Hey, looks like you're the resident crocheting expert. What are you making today?" or one of my old favorites – "I love your tattoos, they are way better than the ones I don't have."

Social Skills — After . . .

Anti-Social, hate crowds, prefer to limit social activity to friends and family. If you could watch a video tape of me in a Costco during rush hour (any hour this place is open pretty much) you will find me flat against a rack or ducking into a quiet section to make sure I don't get hit, hurt, or even spoken to. You will find me eyeing the aisles for empty ones so I can make a clean getaway. If you watch real close you will actually see me jump out of my skin from time to time as I go to extremes to avoid something.

Not one time was I in any real danger, and I really don't know what I was trying to avoid. There are times that I find myself more social than usual, and I do hold up my end of the conversation. However, it is much more likely somebody else will start the conversation. It is still more likely that I will go out of my way to avoid people, even while staying at an RV campground.

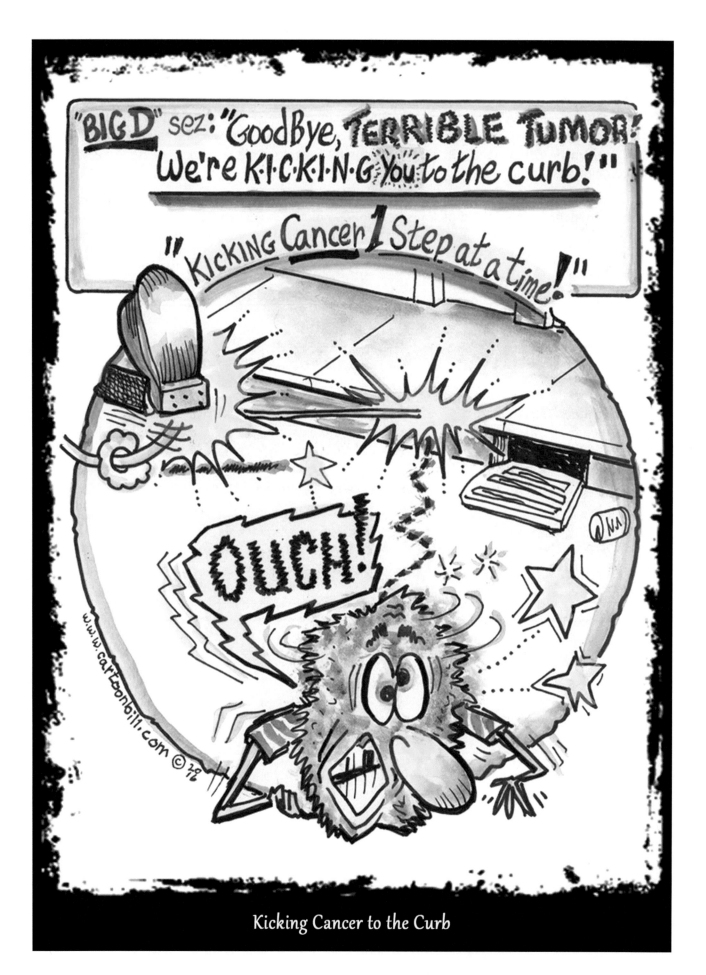

Kicking Cancer to the Curb

Chapter 4

The Diagnosis Process —
You Can't Trust Every Doctor!

"It's a Matter of Trust" by Billy Joel

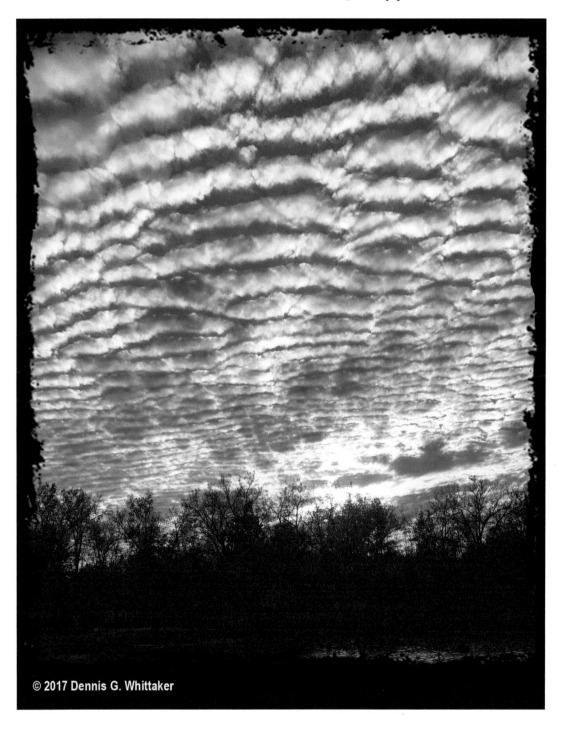

© 2017 Dennis G. Whittaker

We grow up in a society where we are taught to put our trust, and often our lives in the hands of a doctor. After all, they are very dedicated and passionate folks that have invested a ton of cash and time to earn this level of respect.

The question we don't always focus on is this: Are any of the caretakers that worked so hard to earn the certificate on the wall actually good at what they do? I made the mistake of making an assumption in this arena, assuming the qualifications based on said certificate were trustworthy. Oh, and he was on my insurance plan????

Imagine putting this trust in a doctor only to be laughed out of his office after performing a standard test?

All I can say is that I lost 3 months before a proper diagnosis was performed.

I learned that making such an assumption may just change the course of your life!

So, never assume that your caregiver has your best interests at heart or will take the time to perform as we need and expect them to!

Getting The News - Is My Life Insurance Up To Date?

I could be wrong, but I expect that the first thing many folks think about when they are diagnosed with cancer, or any other life-threatening experience, is a bit of a mixed cocktail. For me, I certainly felt like I had a few too many for sure.

Here is the short list of things that bounced through my head: (Please note: After about 5 reviews to date, I realize that I have basically done this project more than once. This is common throughout the process of writing the book. Just a side effect of my brain's inability to remember and process. I have done my best to clean these up throughout the book to ensure a consistent tale. However, the book would not be honest without leaving at least one of these "episodes" intact. My apologies for the duplication)

- ➢ Is my life insurance paid and up to date?
- ➢ Why didn't I buy that damned Cancer Insurance when I could have? (It would have been a terrific investment!)
- ➢ What's for lunch today?
- ➢ How am I gonna pay my bills if I can't work?
- ➢ This is gonna be hard on me, but even harder on my family.
- ➢ I heard about this chemo brain thing, if that's gonna happen to me, I'm out. I would rather die today than live my life being stupid. (I am still alive, and I wouldn't go so far as to call myself stupid, but I am certainly stupider.)
- ➢ This type of cancer can cause all kinds of crazy things, some involving surgery that can affect my ability to eat, talk, and socialize. What exactly did I sign up for here?

It is difficult to describe everything that goes through your mind when you receive a potentially life-threatening diagnosis such as stage 4 cancer. For me, my wife's security was a paramount concern, as was our financial stability going forward as long as I survive. Suddenly, the fine print on life insurance policies became extremely important, and begged answers to these kinds of questions.

- Are my premiums paid?
- Do I have a disability rider?
- Can I cash out some or all of my policy if I have a terminal diagnosis?
- Is it too late to sign up for that cancer policy they offered me two years ago? (Talk about optimism that borders on insanity)
- How many of those "No Questions Asked" Life Insurance Policy's will they sell me?
- Does anyone offer a lifetime cruise around the world for say, $10K or so for my wife and me?

Obviously, you can see where this charming bit of advice is coming from. After you have cancer is not the time to find the right life insurance policy. This is in the same category as "save some money" so if the day comes for you to face these horrifying circumstances, your focus can be on reserving the cruise and not worrying about how you're gonna pay for it!

Truth be told, these are the kinds of things you can and should do to prepare for any of life's little byroads, because you really have no effective way to prepare for the flood of emotions and feelings you will have when you get news like this. Feelings simply don't work that way now do they? If they did, there would be classes in grade school, like "How to deal with the death of a family member, friend, neighbor or celebrity" or "If I am going to die in the next 6 months, what should I feel, and what should I do to prepare for my journey in the afterlife?" Or possibly "If I get to meet Elvis on the other side, what should we talk about, and will I be able to access these questions from Dropbox™ on the other side?"

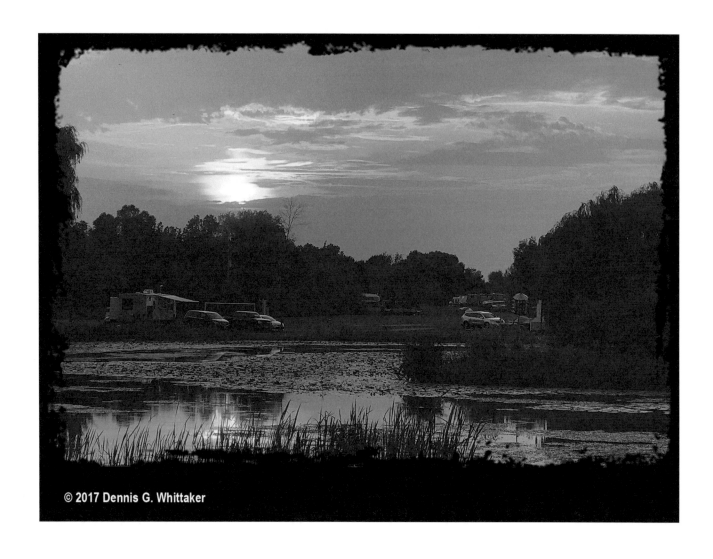

© 2017 Dennis G. Whittaker

"If Today Was Your Last Day" *by Nickleback*

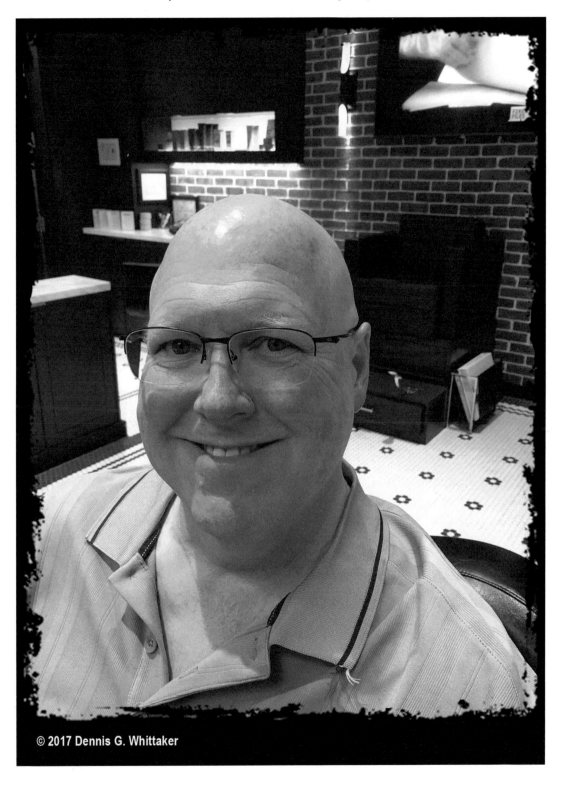

Death has not been a stranger to me. Starting after my family moved from Canada to the Southwest in 1967, our so called "Vacations" were often a trip to Canada to see relatives. Well, to be more accurate, to say goodbye to the dearly departed, and after having flown for 7 hours to get there, we may as well say Hi, have a few beers (root beer for me) and visit the dearly not yet departed, and take in some sights along the way.

My mother often explained that it was important for me to experience this process, so in the unlikely event that someone in the immediate family (huh, what's that?) died, I would be better prepared for it. As the youngest of 9 children, my mother was the perfect teacher of such truths.

I hate to disagree with her, but there was nothing in the world that could have prepared me to see my brother, age 16 when I was 13, get hit by a drunk driver going way too fast around a blind curve. I had to figure out what to do, what to say, and what to do with my bike (AHB comes to mind.) I ended up telling the drunk driver exactly this, in a shaky and very sarcastic voice "Thanks a Lot!", which was later followed by this question to the hostess at the restaurant close to where this took place: "Would it be okay if I park my bike in your lobby, my brother just got hit by a car and I have to go to the hospital right now. I don't want it to get stolen" Once again, I could write another book about this particular chapter of my life. Maybe another time. I have a funeral to go to:(

I enjoyed a reasonably quiet period for a spell, with the exception of a trip or two to Canada, until 1985 came along.

Some chapters in our life we simply can't heal from.

This is the year that my first wife and the first love of my life had her own cancer to deal with. I slept in a recliner at the hospital most every night for what seemed an eternity but was probably about 3 – 6 months before she passed away from pneumonia (rarely does the paperwork state cancer to be the cause of death.) This occurred about 3 months after my Dad died from a massive heart attack, and exactly one month before our first wedding anniversary. This year has shaped so much of who I am today and how I perceive most anything.

Nothing is permanent, and nothing has to make sense. Justice is a word people use to define how they would like to feel about the experiences they have and don't like, but sadly ever do. Saving money and being frugal is pretty much a waste of time, after all, you can't take it with you. If your gonna have any kind of legacy, you better make it quick 'cause you may not be around much longer.

I don't care if my underwear is dirty when I get hit by the bus, but my in-box at work had better be empty!

What I find time to experience is wildly more important to me than how I got there, how nice the accommodations happened to be, and whether the meal was served on a napkin or on the queen's china. First class on an airplane is an illusion. The people sitting next to you will still bitch and complain if they don't like you, find that you're too big for their comfort, or if you dispense one of those silent but deadly bi-labial fricatives (Farts in most circles, Thanks George C:)!

I am not saying here that I want to die or expect to die anytime soon. Let's just say that I have realized that my goal for the rest of my days is to enjoy the simple things, catch people doing things right and rewarding them for it somehow, and to know, when my time does come, I will be at peace with myself, my life and the comfort to know that my in-box is indeed empty.

B5 *Sleeping — Before . . .*

Sleep? What's all this noise about sleep?

On a really good night, I could sleep about 6 hours. It was usually 4 or 5.

This started to change when I had cancer and didn't know it yet, as I started to nod off any time after about 7:30 pm.

I was also more likely to sleep till about 6.

Sleeping — After . . .

I now sleep comfortably from about 10 at night till about 7:30 in the morning. I may get up for a nature call, play a game or two on my phone, then back to bed for another round.

Afternoon naps don't happen every single day anymore, but I tend to get a 2-4 hour nap 3-5 times a week.

As much as I try to manage stress every day, there is simply no avoiding it altogether. The day following an especially stressful day will all but guarantee a four-hour recovery nap for the next 2-3 days.

It is now about 14 months since my last cancer treatment, so it seems to be a new way of life, and not so much an Artifact:)

Chapter 5

"Don't Stop Thinking About Tomorrow" *by Fleetwood Mac*

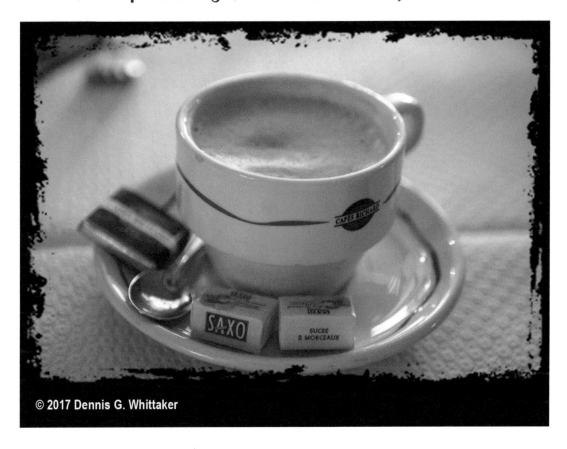

© 2017 Dennis G. Whittaker

37

Just a couple of days ago, I was working on all kinds of very important projects. After all, my next bonus was in sight, and good luck keeping me from making that happen, right?

While the desire and drive to make every day as normal as before, and the focus on these monetary goals is still very much alive, the priorities shift. Everything happens so fast, it is more like I am watching a movie and not experiencing my own life. The sets are changed, the script is updated. New characters audition and are rewarded heavily for their roles as your new team of life-saving medical professionals gather to solve your problems.

Before chemo, they install a "Medi-Port." This clever little device gets installed in your main artery going into your heart, and makes it easier, faster, and less painful to hook up your IV's to this amazing and "Life Saving Medicine" (reference to the episode of Archer where he is diagnosed with cancer a few times.)

Please note: Life Saving Cancer Medications actually kill off a lot of things. While the intention is purely to kill off cancer cells, it also kills white blood cells, brain cells, motivational cells, being alert and awake cells as well as the desire to live through all this, cells.

Some things in life are entertaining, kinda. It was peculiar to me that many of the folks that took my blood were not aware of this amazing thing in my chest. It turned out to be my personal responsibility to ensure that this expensive device and related installation expense was honored as often as possible.

The process went kinda like this - (this is exaggerated in hopes of tickling your funny bone, and not to insult the loving and hardworking phlebotomists that worked tirelessly on my behalf.)

- Needle Person: "We need to take 77 vials of blood from you for testing before your next treatment. Please roll up your sleeve"
- Me: "I have a Medi-Port right here that cost thousands of dollars, and is easier, faster and less painful than having you poke me 1 to 6 times to find an appropriate dispensing tube inside of my arm. Would you like to use it?"
- Needle Person: "Oh, you have a Medi-port?"
- Me: "DUH!"
- Needle Person: "Do you want me to use that instead of poking you an unknown number of times in your arm?"
- Me: "DUH!"
- Needle Person: "Let me look at your chart to see if it is okay to use this wildly expensive and convenient thingy."
- Me: "FM!" Okay, back to the movie set where filming will continue:

The set of my office at work (desk, computer, telephone, printer, chair, filing cabinet, chairs for 1 or 2 victims to be "Whittaker'ed" (yup, this became a verb back in my working days. It was a blessing and/ or curse for all who were exposed to it.))

This set has been donated to someone that can put it to good use, as I am no longer able to manage it. The new set in my life includes an entire host of offices, test equipment, medical equipment, needles, drugs, nuclear medicine, et al.

The usual cast of fellow workers, customers, and the goofy guy at the coffee shop have all been replaced with doctors, nurses, technicians, and the folks that love answering phones and making appointments.

The uniforms are so different as well. No more suits, ties, company shirts or logoed apparel. Well, the doctors still dress that way, but everyone else is wearing scrubs, and those wildly comfortable shoes.

They all did their best to make me feel comfortable and well cared for. If these folks are just in it for the money, they all deserve an Academy award, as I never once had that nasty feeling that they were doing anything other than doing what they loved and getting paid for it!

B8 Balance — Before . . .

No gymnast, but could stay on feet all the time.

Balance — After . . .

Serious Balance issues finally resolved through Physical Therapy. After going through a battery of 7 tests, the only thing left to cause the problem was an issue with my personal CPU (Brain.)

Walking Calculator, Deep Thinker, Could Solve Most Any Problem In my Head with as many process steps as needed to ensure accuracy, quality and repeatability. Developed / Engineered Many Complex Software Solutions.

I made more money over the years doodling engineering drawings or software ideas on a napkin during a lunch conversation. A doodle here and there and everyone was on the same page. It's not that I was some amazing artist, quite the opposite most of the time. This is why I tried to surround myself with folks that could see through the scratches of all this and join me in knowing that it can be done, and that we can get it done.

Maybe my next book will get into some details of some of these things, but for now, feel free to Google these: "PanelCrafters™ – CADBlox™, the brain trust that others grew into WEBlox™, Easy-Linx™ and Kettle Chefs™ to name a few ideas that started on a napkin.

Math Skills — After . . .

Love these calculator thingies, can now solve any problem so long as it is only a single step solution. Can no longer understand how to modify or create new sections in the data-base program I designed and programed from nothing. It tied 5 independent systems together in one place that allowed for a view of the business that couldn't be found anywhere else. The ability to immediately zoom in on productivity and profits from the company, to the division, to the team and all the way down to the individual honed an amazing way to constantly and consistently improve the business.

The day came where I had spent 30 hours working on a single report for the new quarter, and it wasn't right. Pre-Cancer, I updated, created and launched the entire suite of programs and reports in about a day. This was the day I knew, without question or reservation, that I was truly disabled. My email to my boss and the folks in HR was one of the most difficult times for me to hit the send button.

Chapter 6

Halloween Anyone?
Getting Ready for Radiation?

"Witch Hunt" (Part III of Fear) by Rush

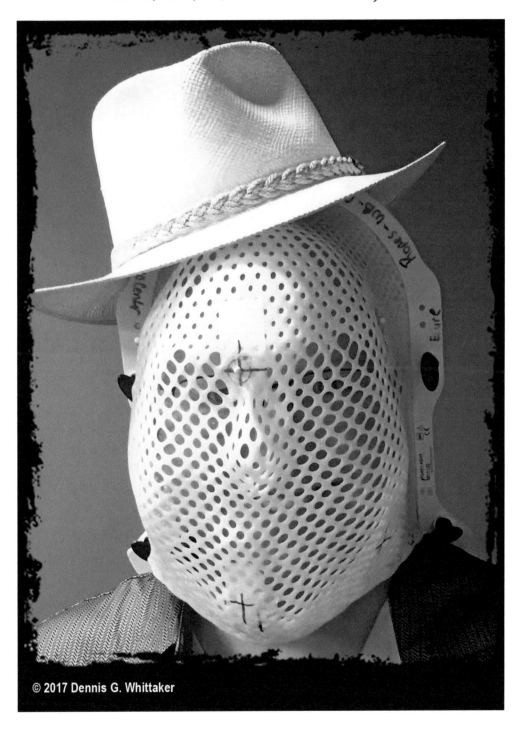

© 2017 Dennis G. Whittaker

I have worn various Halloween costumes over the years. Most of them reasonably inexpensive. The most expensive one was the gorilla costume that I rented for $75 back in college in hopes of getting a gal to go ape with me, which is simply $75 I will never get back.

For those of us that need radiation treatments to our head or neck, we get to wear a very expensive costume indeed. It is made of a special material that softens in hot water. You lay on a machine that is identical to the one they use for the actual radiation treatments down the hall. This funky green mesh is pushed down over your face and clicks into the table. Then you wait for it to cool, which will hold its new shape.

Turns out, the most critical aspect of this process is the tiny little dot they put on it that is used to register the amazing machine that will perform the "35 Daily Zaps" (next chapter please.)

Unfortunately for me, there was an issue with said dot. This is a bad thing, as the next step is to perform a dry run to ensure that everything is properly set up and good to go. In my case, it wasn't set up properly and became a no-go instead. This pushed this precisely timed process back a week or two. At that time, I still had enough brain cells to be concerned about the mathematical circumstances of this delay.

In short, cancer cells divide and multiply much more efficiently than rabbits. The goal of the radiation, and the reason it is critical not to miss a single appointment, is that each session will kill off a certain number of these cells. Within 24 hours, while feeling somewhat disrespected and therefore unwelcomed, they will do their very best to reproduce in order to replace all of their kin that died earlier that day. It's a major project by the time they respect the dead, find a mate, do their thing, etc. etc. etc., You get the picture.

The Radiation Oncologist is very good at this little war game, and somehow knows how many of these he needs to kill each day to keep up with this crazy level of procreation. So, if you attend all 35 sessions and remember not to move for the few seconds of the process, the ability of these cancer cells to live in this never-ending orgy they call life, will cease, and you will become cancer free, or "In Remission."

Mind you, this is no promise that you will remain cancer free. Lots of percentages come up for discussion based on your cancer type, age, how much you drink, how much you smoke, and of course how many of those grease filled spongy snack thingy's (Twinkies®) you eat every day. They will all play into which side of the 40-90% chance of survival they discuss.

Key point here, works like this. Surviving is just that. It means that you will be able to take more breaths, think more thoughts (hopefully) and adapt to the new you as you do your best to Live long and prosper! (Spock from Star Trek) It does not mean that life will ever be the same again. The treatment process will change you, possibly in many ways.

Your dedication and ability to manage what you have left to work with, will define the quantity and quality of your life going forward. As I like to say - "Gotta breathe, may as well enjoy it!

Chapter 7

35 Daily Zaps —
Like Swallowing Boiling Oil

"That's Gonna Leave A Scar" by *Sixx AM*

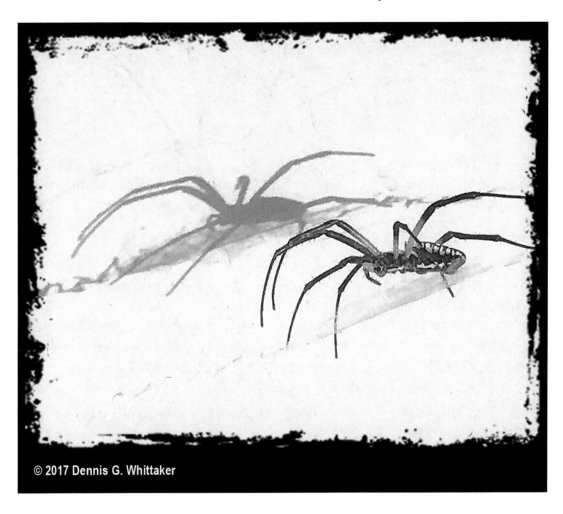

© 2017 Dennis G. Whittaker

It all starts out harmless enough it seems. These folks are glad to see you and are thankful to have an opportunity to put their hard-earned talents to good use.

Somewhere around this time, you start to understand how this entire process is engineered and managed. It goes like this:

➢ Don't tell 'em too much of the story all at once, or they will run away!!!!!

So, the story unfolds as you go.

At first, it is a couple of very simple things you need to go through, then all will be normal once again.

- Testing   - Radiation

- Chemo   - Recovery

Each of these things occur in exactly that order, only there is a lot more to the story as it turns out. This story is unique to each person, their health, where they live and, of course, how many of those spongy sugary things consumed.

In any event, here is the rest of MY story:

❖ **Testing** – This stage alone would never ever be used on a person that doesn't already have cancer, as it will likely give you cancer.
  - Well, actually, we are going to run some radio-active dye into your body so it can light up the areas where your cancer is hanging out.

  - Then, we are gonna sit you in a room with 2' thick concrete walls for an hour, because we don't want anybody else to glow in the dark.

  - Then we are gonna ask you to lay perfectly still for a few (like 20 or 30) minutes, while we do the actual scan.

  - Repeat as needed throughout your cancer treatments to validate the results.

❖ **Chemo** – Some of these observations come from what the doctors tell you, others are what you learn on your own as you go through this.
  - We will have you come in every 21 days for chemo. It is a simple concoction of 3 drugs, which are all designed to kill off human tissue. But don't worry, we have done our very best to design them to kill mostly the bad cancerous ones. Any negative effect on other human tissue is not intended or desired. Please refer to any one of the more than 374 pages of the permissions you have signed to realize this: "It is What it is!:"

  - By the way, these drugs will make you nauseous, so we will be injecting you with some anti-nausea meds, then send you home with pills to stave it off between sessions.

  - Oh yeah, we are also gonna send you home with another kind of chemo, so you will have to babysit this wildly fun and expensive fanny pack that has an IV pump and special drugs.

- OH, and Oh yeah, we are gonna need for you to get this tiny little $7K box attached to your arm, so in exactly 27 hours, we will be able to inject you with something that is designed to make your white blood cells happy (happier at least) so they will continue to fight a good fight for you, our latest "VIP" (Short for : "Very Immunologically-Challenged Patient".) They even gave me a VIP card so they will know what to do with me if and when I need to go to the emergency room.

- Oh, OH, and Oh yeah, you may lose some hair along the way (not to get too personal about this, but let's just say that the boys feel kinda strange when they're bald)

- And by the by, you may or may not find yourself losing your temper. My wife learned this quickly: "It is recommended that children under the age of 100 stay clear of Dennis at any time that his face is red, his fists are clenched, and his mouth is swollen open, as what is left of his brain tries to find the exact words to describe exactly how much this little episode will potentially destroy anyone stupid enough to stick around for the violence and profanity that is surely heading their way, very, very soon!"

❖ *Radiation*

- The oncologist warns you about what you're going to go through by simply stating "Let me know if you need any pain meds as you go through this." This is like saying something along the lines of "Let me know if you need a towel to dry off after you fall off the Golden Gate Bridge, 'cause you may be a tad wet!

- The first week is pretty much a no brainer. It's almost like they are just getting you in the groove of the daily commute to the cancer center.

- The second week, you get tired all the time, but no biggie.

- Week three,,,,,,,,Mmm, what did I sign up for here? Can I get a refund? I really don't like this amusement park so much anymore. And by the way, where is that guy's phone number who promised he could get me the good meds.

- Sleep is good, yes, I really should just take a liiittttle na,,,,,,,,,,p,,,,,,,.

- Week four, mmmm, this is weird, I coulda swore I cracked them eggs before I scrambled em up in the fry pan. Why does it hurt so much to swallow them? Oh, I know, they need more cheese next time, got it!!!!

- Week Five, Week Six and Week Seven – Please leave a message at the beep, as I am currently on the Fentanyl Cloud contemplating if I ever really wanna come back to reality. Reality hasn't been very nice to me lately, and my wife would be much better off financially from the life insurance proceeds. (I can relax about this, as I was in fact, up to speed on my previously mentioned premium payments.)

- Day one, Week Eight: WHAT! I was told this was a seven-week process! WTF!!@@!!

Oh, and bye the bye, the radiation is just really picking up steam. "Sorry, I didn't realize that you were expecting a reprieve after the treatments are over. The next two weeks will be a living hell. Would you like some more of the Fentanyl patches to get you through?" This was mid-August, and I was on Fentanyl until late November.

So, what else is there to say about this? You end up on autopilot for a few months, nothing exciting to report, outside of the hope that this phase will be both over and successful as soon as possible. A man can only live on cheese and eggs for so long, right?

Did I mention that I was asked to gain 40 pounds prior to the radiation, in order to be able to live through the process? So now, I am in remission, Yeah!, but I am also back in the old swing of eating too much and not exercising enough. The demons of cholesterol et al. are back for a visit.

B7 Decision Making — Before . . .

Pre-Cancer, I was ridiculously confident on any subject where I could "feel" that I was correct. I was wildly competitive and worked myself to the bone to make it happen.
I challenged people to grow to their full potential and watched them as they learned, earned and accomplished things they didn't know anything about before we met.

Seeing someone I hired buy their first new car, new house, have a baby, earn a promotion or become successful filled me with a kind of pride and joy that continues to lighten my load as concerns about my legacy grows.

I hired some of the most talented and intelligent people. But this isn't about me really, it's all about how these folks were willing to learn new things, see the world a different way, and make something of themselves.

Decision Making — After . . .

Let's just say that self-confident would no longer be the word I use to describe myself.

Let's see now:

I don't drive, as I can't process the information in front of me quickly enough to slam on the brakes, take the correct exit, or to remember to order extra hot fudge at the Baskin Robbins drive through.

My wife has come to understand that it is now her job to order our meal at a restaurant. This solves three problems at one time.

1. A decision can be made in a reasonable time frame.

2. We can share a meal, which is indeed good for the budget.

3. We can share a meal, which is indeed good for our health.

Many of my decisions should have been left to others. (Please see the anecdote about having to fire myself on Page 53:)

The only thing more stressful to me than making a quick decision is to manage the results and consequences, and costs for the ones I make.

Chapter 8

The Guilt, Anxiety, and Loss of Control

"F**CK YOU" by Lily Allen

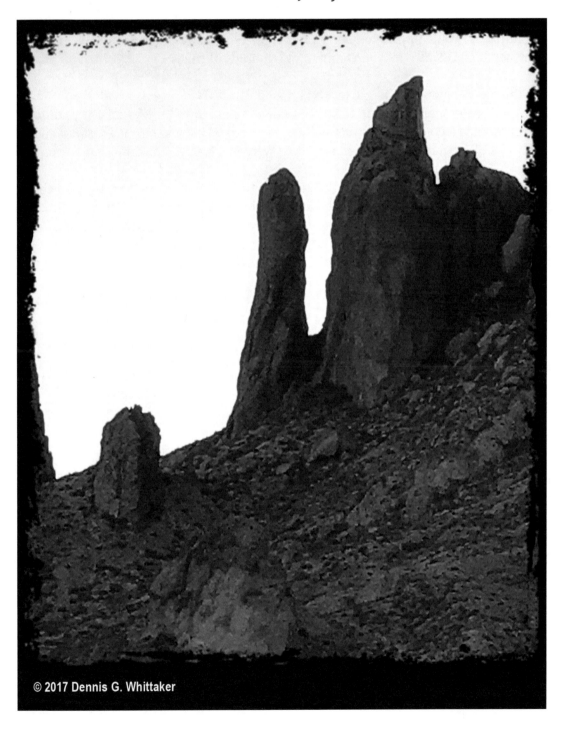

© 2017 Dennis G. Whittaker

Okay, Enough of the Happy Horseshit!

At this moment in time, life sucks, IT REALLY Sucks! This next section will not be pleasant, so please don't expect it to be. For the historians, this writing begins at 8:11 pm on Saturday, September 23, 2017.

I have had two completely nasty and unique headaches today. The words "FUCK ME!!! (FM going forward!) have been on the tip of my tongue since about 6:45 am. It reminds me of the episode of South Park, that was all about "They are going to say "Shit" on TV." The show had a counter on it, for every time the word was used, some # of hundreds of times. My version of the show, "the real-life story of Dennis G Whittaker" would have a counter on it to track how many times I said FM, either out loud or screaming inside my head, also in some number of hundreds of times.

Here's the thing. I am literally allergic to stress. Good Stress, Bad Stress, it's all the same. I tell people this from time to time, designed to be a warning system to folks. My hope is to diffuse what can and will likely become a complete rant that will cut even the tallest and strongest of my audience into a pile of bubbling fools trying to understand why they were just hit by a tsunami of epic proportions.

I am quite confident that the folks at the generator repair shop that I went to this past February still have the FM sound ringing in their ears, and have added special training classes from time to time, providing each employee with the skills to recognize anyone showing the signs of a stress allergy, what is going to happen soon, when to put on the OSHA approved hearing protection, and exactly how to bring this asshole back to a somewhat normal state of breathing.

I can always tell the folks that haven't been to this lifesaving class because they always say the same stupid thing when I tell them that I am allergic to stress. Hold on, here it comes,, "Aren't we all!"

In mathematical terms, my reaction to stress is roughly 1.2 million times more ferocious and negative than the average person living at the time of this writing. I mention average, as this is no claim to having the largest or worst allergy of this kind, as I am sure others have an even harder time dealing with the daily ins and outs of making it through the day.

I know what you're thinking: "Man, this guy must have literally lived through an entire country song in a single day! He lost his wife, dog, girlfriend, truck, job, sense of self, reason to live, fishing boat, last cold brew, and his best friend (due to the new relationships said best friend is now enjoying with his now ex-wife AND girlfriend,) all in a single day! OMFingG!!!!!

Not even close. Here is a reasonably complete list of what made this day so ever worthy of a total mental and emotional meltdown:

1. I dropped a nice stack of plastic support plates for my trailer and had to stack them up again.   (FM Count =1)

2. My wife wanted me to dump the sewer tanks, total time approx. 5.32 minutes. (FM Count =2)

3. The campground we were headed to didn't answer and sent me to VM. (FM Count = 3)

4. The amazing and exquisite design my friend and I came up with to hold my portable waste tank to the back of my trailer fell off yesterday. (Okay, some of today's stress carried over from yesterday.) This design occupied my thoughts for days and weeks, then took another few days and many hours with my friend at various hardware stores to perfect. Just 6 minutes before a kindly driver pulled us to the side of the road to let us know that we were dragging it around behind us, I had proudly told my wife that all was well with this, and how we had come up with the very best and most affordable design known to man. (Total FM count is now over 312 and counting)

Today is a new day. I know this because that calendar indicates it is now Tuesday October 2nd, 2017, which is a different date than was listed above. These calendar thingies are awesome!

Back to today, which was a great day, well, at least it was until it wasn't. I was back on my horse tackling for the n-teenth time, the project mentioned above. Proudly prepared to set the record straight with the new perfected design, #56.5. It was time to go outside, say hello to a perfect day, and kick this particular project to the curb, so to speak.

As I step out of the trailer onto the step, I find a major flaw in my new design. I missed the most important step of the new project, which of course was the step outside my trailer. Missing a step, as most folks have experienced, is a bad idea, and may end badly. For me, it was one of those shiner things, on my knee instead of my eye, some nice scrapes and scratches and some very sore toes.

What, you may be thinking, what does this have to do with this chapter, which is supposed to be about Guilt, Anxiety, and the Loss of Control?

This is how this story breaks down, in mathematical terms:

1. Falling down for no good reason is clearly an indicator that I had a total and complete loss of control. This counts for 27% of the reason this story fits into this chapter.

2. Laying stunned on the ground made me feel stupid and inadequate (Please see Chapter "10", B7 Decision Making — Anecdote . . .) for more on this vicious circle. Feeling this way, makes me anxious, mostly because I now have zero confidence in what I was going to do, as I haven't even made it to step 1 without failing miserably. This counts for 37.5% of the reason this story fits into this chapter.

3. However, the number 1 reason, which accounts for approximately 100% of the reason this fits into this chapter is the overwhelming guilt this 3 second experience has caused. My wife has her hands full. She is responsible for pretty much everything these days. She does all the driving, cooks most of the meals, does all of the laundry, feeds and brushes the dog, reminds me to brush my teeth and take a shower, and exactly 1003 other things, if listed, would take up this entire book. The one thing that overshadows her every day is her concern about me and my welfare.

I have become a full-time job, which she somehow manages to stay on top of while managing the suite of full time jobs mentioned above. She is constantly looking out for me and thinks about what she can do to keep me safe, healthy and upright. In a matter of these few seconds, I have managed to put that part of her job on high alert. This will affect her every minute of every day, as she feels there had to be something she could have done to protect me from myself. (Good luck with that honey!)

Later in the evening, I take Hado for a walk. A leisurely stroll, lighted by an almost full moon, and the light from my cell phone. It turned out to be an unusually long walk. As my wife had just patched me up with a box of band-aids a couple of hours ago, it is easy to see why she was concerned when we hadn't come back in a timely fashion. She jumped in the car and drove all over the campground looking for me, fully expecting that once again, I had found a way to get hurt. While I was fine when she found us, she was beside herself, realizing that she had gone through this entire process for no other reason other than that she loved me enough to care about me in this way.

So, this is where the guilt comes in. I fully realize the burden that my wife has these days. Well, maybe not. One can't really understand another's experience any ole way. However, the fact remains that there are many factors in our life today that she has been sentenced to, from our finances, to the cancer, to the artifacts. These are all things that are uniquely mine, but are things that she must deal with 24/7. I would trade anything to take this burden away from her, so she could enjoy every moment of every day in peace.

No worries about money, no worries that I will fall and get hurt, forget to look both ways before crossing the street or an entire list of things that folks of retirement age need not be responsible for.

This situation weighs heavy in my heart, and that weight can be measured in guilt. I believe this to be a somewhat useless emotion, especially under the circumstances, but wouldn't it be irresponsible to not take the time to understand how this chapter of our lives has affected her?

This is what actual empathy must feel like. It isn't something I am doing to earn a bonus, it is a genuine concern regarding these circumstances. The AHB side of me must have taken a hard hit during the fall, as this is pretty new to me. It is difficult and overwhelming to feel this way.

Speaking of empathy, today was the day the Las Vegas shooting was in the news. 59 good folks shot down, and 500+ that sustained injuries. In the past, news like this was like watching a movie or reading a book for me. It really didn't affect me outside of the knowledge that this person was a mess and shoulda been locked up some time ago. This is not how the shooting affected me today. I have been moody about it since I first heard about it. It has shaken me to the core and have found myself to be dumbfounded with how this came to be, why nobody noticed how he managed to get 13 suitcases with 23 rifles and God knows how many rounds of ammo up to the 32nd floor of a building that has enough security to protect Fort Knox.

I can't begin to say how much I want to be there to comfort those that have been directly affected by this real-world horror movie.

But it is better if I stay here and avoid any steps. No need to become a burden to others and take away the support they need for themselves.

A note to my Psychologist. I believe this to be the saddest and funniest thing I have ever written.

10/5/2017

Hi Doc!

I had to fire myself today, cause this guy is completely incompetent. His heart is in the right place, but he just can't complete a single project properly. He has cost me thousands in raw materials and tools. It's great that he is willing to work for free but I can't afford to keep him on any longer.

I have hired and fired my share of folks over the years, and letting someone go is still difficult for me, but this is the toughest one yet. His resume looked so promising, and I just couldn't see a downside to giving him a chance.

Back to the drawing board. I can always go to that 6th grade technical school to find a candidate capable of these simple projects.

I think I will go drown myself in a tub of Dragons Milk (a beer stored in bourbon barrels) in hopes it will clear my conscience for firing this guy!

FUCK ME!!!!!!

(P.S., This is not a suicide note, just my way of trying to come to terms that I really need to quit trying to create and invent things. I have spent dozens of hours trying to design new steps for the trailer because I am not comfortable with the plastic ones now in use. They just don't feel safe to me.

The fact that I missed a step a couple of days ago and banged the crap out of my knee drove me even harder to figure this one out. At this moment I am in the same place on this project as if I had been in a coma the entire time.

It will likely be one of many unsolved puzzles (spelled "FRUSTRATIONS") that are now defining who I am and what I will be for the rest of my days.)

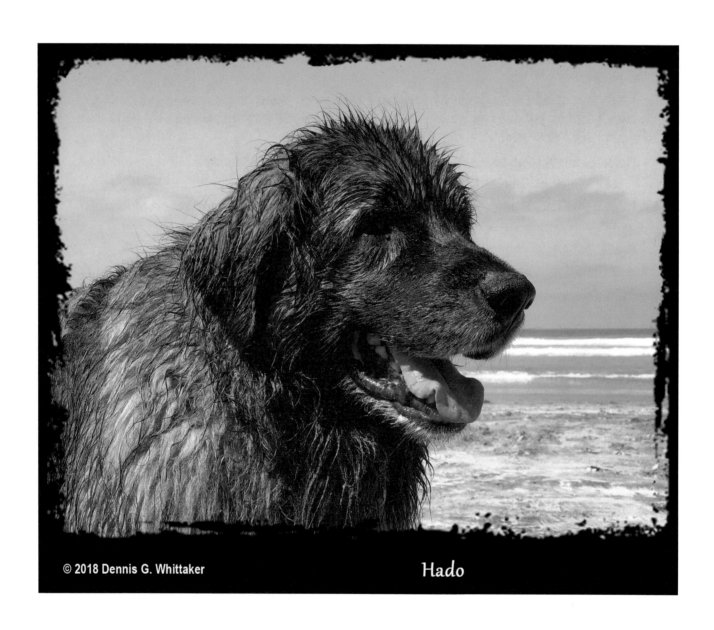

Hado

Chapter 9

The Fentanyl Days

"Does Anybody Really Know What Time it is?" by *Chicago*

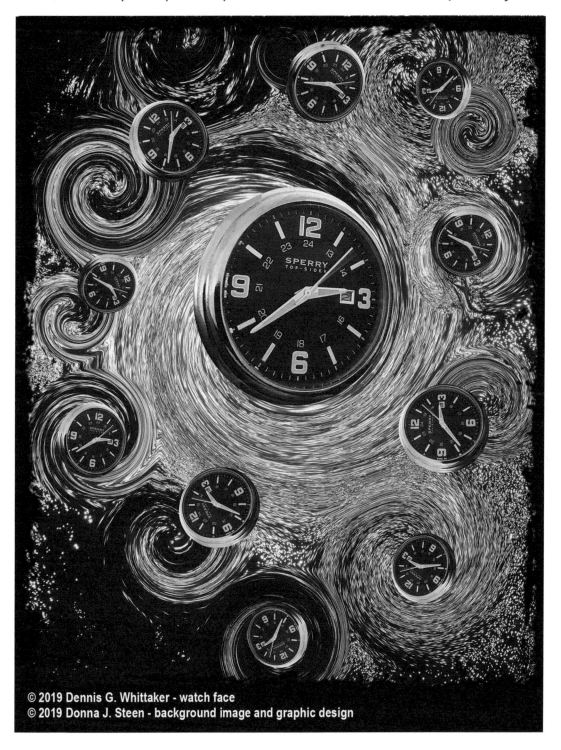

If memory serves, which clearly at this point, it does not, I started using Fentanyl Patches sometime in late July or early August of 2016 (To loosely quote Steve Martin: "Definitely not before July!")

As mentioned previously, getting radiation has an effect similar to swallowing boiling oil, which I expect is very painful indeed. Fentanyl is great for anyone who has experienced either. It is now the leading cause of death by overdose in the United States. For me, I just needed to hear the word "Opiate" to let me know that this was serious stuff (50 to 100X more powerful than Heroin, they say.) As my entire life history for illegal drugs included less than 1/3rd of a joint, I had no idea what to expect. One would think that my brain's ability to truly experience color would drive right past the current "X" Millions available on our cell phone, right? Not at all.

Mostly, I slept. Waking long enough to hug my wife, brush my teeth, (yup, you're right, my priorities were backwards) eat some eggs with cheese, go back to bed, get told to get up and "Take A Shower For God's Sake! Take said shower and then lay down to sleep through another rerun of Archer or the Murdoch Mysteries.

When I found that going back to work wasn't gonna work for me, I got approval to work from home. As a workaholic, I expected these days to be gloriously productive, as I would be able to work uninterrupted, any hour of the day, any day of the week. Frankly, I was miserably wrong here.

I don't know when the Fentanyl Days blended into the MNCD Days, and it really doesn't matter. The fact is that a normal hour of productivity slowly moved from one to 1 ½ to 2, to 3 to 4, etc.

It can now take me 20-30 hours to accomplish some version of the objective, as demonstrated here:

9/24/2017:

Had a bit of a crazy week.

I worked on a project to mount something on the back of my RV. This may have taken 1 1/2 hours precancer and would have worked better than expected.

This one took me 6 designs, 20 hours or more and 4 trips to Home Depot, all to have the damn thing fall off a week later.

Somewhere in the book I reference a time that my ego was sulking in the corner of the room. I only wish I could remember which corner, so I could find him and encourage him to join me again.

In the fits and spurts that I was awake, I was worried (strange for Mr. Teflon™. What the hell is going on with this feeling?) that I would become addicted to this drug. I shared my concerns with my oncologist, who laughed lovingly, and told me that I had little or nothing to be concerned about. He said that when you take Fentanyl to deal with this kind of physical pain it rarely ends up being a problem. The addictions come from those using it for recreational purposes.

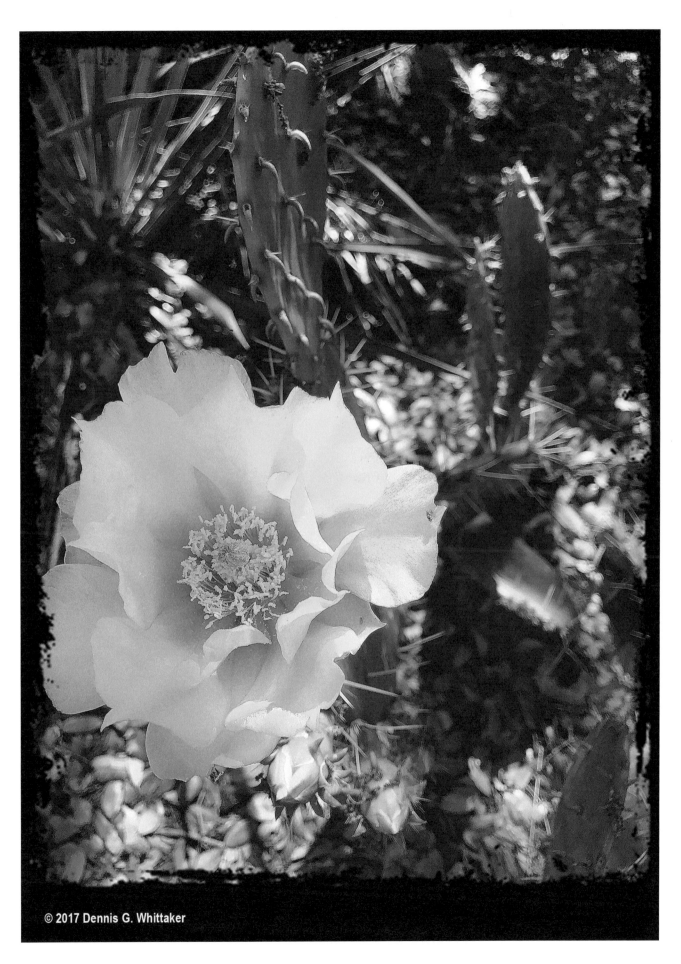

One day, maybe late October, I had a very vivid and freaky colorful dream. This was my clue to start cutting back on my patches. I took this clue seriously, and 3 weeks later I was done with this chapter of my life (and this book)

PS: I have a few of these patches left. Anyone interested in purchasing the remaining stock can place a bid at "crazycolorfuldreams.com."

PLEASE NOTE:

Any and all costs associated with the conquences of this highly illegal transaction and all legal costs and expenses incurred on behalf of the seller shall be paid by the purchaser. He/She/They also agree to be a surrogate prisoner, if needed, to take my place in any prison the judge deems reasonable for such a crime.

AKA – These things are not for sale, EVER!!!!

Chapter 10

The Recovery

"Maybe It's Time" *by Sixx AM*

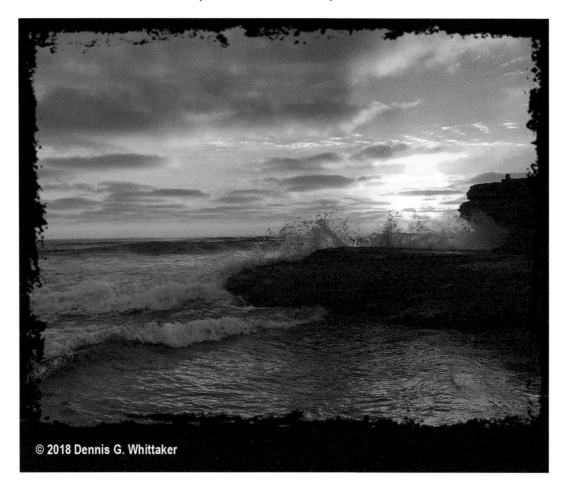

© 2018 Dennis G. Whittaker

They say there is no such thing as a recovered alcoholic, gambler, dieter, football fan / soccer fan et al.: It is my belief that there is also no such thing as a "Recovered Cancer Patient."

Some of us die (Damned Cancer) which is the most extreme lack of recovery, and some of us go back to a very normal life, only cancer free.

However, we all live in the shadows and fear of what may come roaring back once again, only this time it may not go away so easily. (Easy, as in trying to pull a freight train up a hill with an HO scale engine.)

Some of us (as in you, not me, that's for sure) manage this easily, while others will be looking over our shoulder and under the bed as we do everything possible to hide from the ugly monster that created these real-world nightmares. Nightmares that make the very best horror movies that have ever come out of Hollywood seem like comedies.

This is a fear that you can't run away from. For me, everything I experience is akin to looking through a new set of glasses. These glasses range the full gamut, from too weak, so everything is blurry all the time, to too strong, so everything is blurry all the time, to the fancy rose colored ones, where we talk ourselves into believing that life is perfect just the way it is now.

For obvious reasons, I prefer the Rose-Colored pair. It allows me to continue to focus on the optimism that there is soooo much more to live, love and cherish.

This isn't a Rose-Colored vision but is actually 100% true and accurate.

The main thing the Rose-Colored pair does for me is to help color the ugly things that have happened and will continue to happen going forward to find the courage to go forward another day, and to conquer all my demons (yup, I am human after all, so cancer is not alone in my den of demons.)

So, now that all that ugliness is out of my system, let's look at the brave new world, which is called "remission." This is kind of a combo of the "guilt, anxiety, and loss of control" chapter tossed in with the new world we call recovery.

As of this writing, it has been 14 months since the end of all cancer treatments. Life, one would expect, would be kinda back to normal,,, or NOT! Now, while dealing with life's various artifacts, coming up next there is a brand-new layer of guilt and anxiety to go along with it.

Out of the blue, I continue to blow up at very good people for little or no reason. (Please see the previous reference to the vicious circle that follows this.) This process completely drains me, as it feels (and smells) like my brain synapses are frying throughout this process. My propensity to feel and be stupid and reasonably useless are confirmed once more. My ability to think, manage stress and have a truly exceptional attitude have all gone AWOL for a spell, until a few of these burnt out bridges can be brought back on-line.

Going through this is draining. I sleep even more, eat too much, worry about where this is all headed. Then I grow a pair and tell myself to quit focusing on these things that can't be changed or affected in a positive way by giving them the power to control my every thought and decision.

This of course, is empowering. For a spell, I feel invincible, so I take on a little project, and everything is now perfect, as in perfectly back to the way things used to be, which is the way things are supposed to be, right? This is a temporary source of relief. Yup, your right! Now feeling invincible, I take on another project, then another. Then, within two hours of each other, these new projects both fail. MISERABLY! This seems wildly unlikely, as I am back to my old self again, right? WRONG!

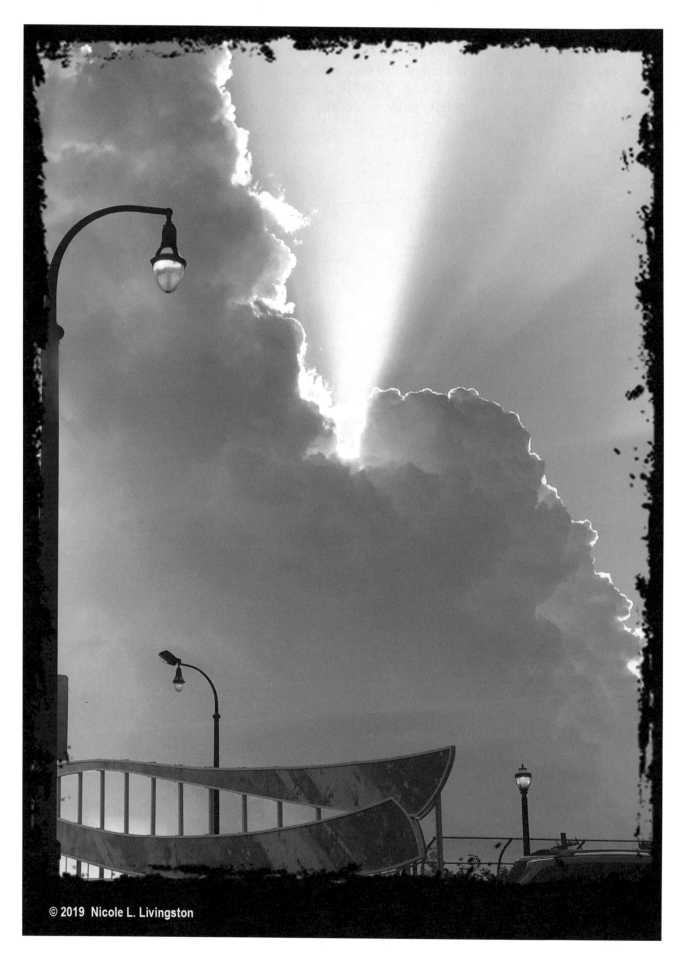

Chapter 11

The Artifacts — AKA
The Side Effects

"Marion's Theme" from Raiders of the Lost Ark *by John Williams*

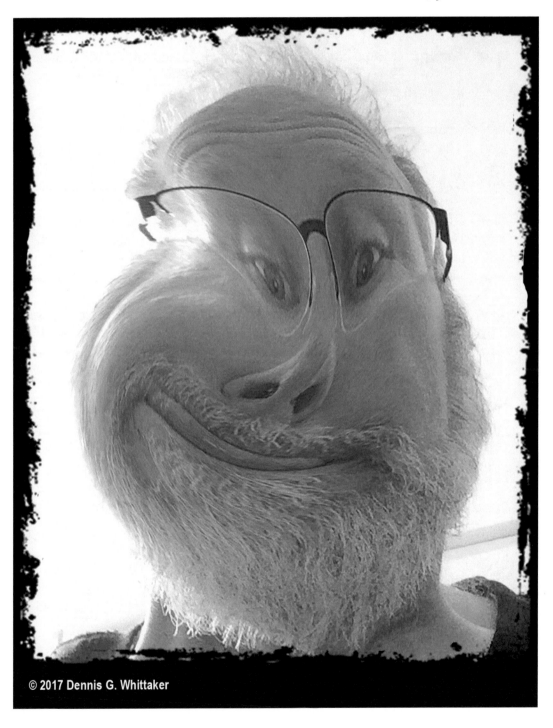

Some folks name their cars, navigation systems and other stuff. Me, I decided to name and categorize all the various side effects from my cancer treatments as Artifacts! This word brings up all kinds of interesting thoughts from movies like "Raiders of the Lost Ark," which romanticize some interesting concepts.

To support my naming convention, per Merriam Webster, here is the definition of the word ar·ti·fact:[1]

\ˈärt-ə-,fakt\   noun

1. an object made by a human being, typically an item of cultural or historical interest.

   "gold and silver artifacts"

   synonyms: relic, article;
                     handiwork

   "hundreds of unidentified artifacts are stored in numerous rooms beneath the museum"

2. something observed in a scientific investigation or experiment that is not naturally present but occurs as a result of the preparative or investigative procedure. "wide spread tissue infection may a technical artifact"

I am comfortable with this definition, as I am a human being (or am I???) I consider myself to be somewhat worldly and cultured, and my ego believes and hopes that I will leave this planet with a legacy of sorts that will reflect favorably on my time here on planet earth. Weaving its own way into history that is of interest to at least one other person.

Of course, the entire process of cancer awareness and treatments are wildly scientific, and if nothing else, cancer could easily be defined as a "widespread tissue infection."

So, let me start with my brain issues.

My memory is pretty well shorted out in a number of ways. It has adapted similarly to how folks that go blind but can now hear 10X better.

---

1. "artifact." Merriam-Webster.com. Merriam-Webster, 2017

I can't do any real math in my head anymore whilst I used to be somewhat of a walking calculator. However, today, I would be a much better player of games like "Trivia."

- If I look up a phone number on the web, which for some stupid reason isn't linked to make a call, it will take me 3 times to enter it incorrectly, and two to three more times to get the numbers in the right order. However, well, I can't remember what I was going to say here. Go figure, right?

- Multi-Tasking is now a complete joke to me. I now have at least 20 separate to-do lists. I don't really know where they are. Some are on scraps of paper, others in one app or another on my phone, and yet others are neatly tucked away in some notebooks. Of course, I can't remember where I put them, or what notes I stored in any of them. Basically, if something important needs to be completed, I need to stop everything, and I mean EVERYTHING! To make a calendar note or alarm to remind me. It helps if I write it down really quick, 'cause I will likely forget what was so important by the time I find my phone, open the app, and start making an entry.

Multi-Tasking is a good launchpad to discuss the vicious circle of how little resistance I now have to stress. It goes kinda like this:

1. Many things make me feel stupid and inadequate.

   a. Not remembering common words.

   b. Unable to add 2 numbers that involve carrying a 1 as I will forget what the 1 has the honor of being added to. Now I need to have my calculator app at the ready all the time.

   c. Re-doing the same one-hour project 5 times before getting it right, with each attempt lasting 3-30 hours. One project took me four trips to the hardware store, each over 1.5 hours long before finally obtaining the 6 parts I needed to complete the project. Four months later I finally completed this very complicated task of adding 6 feet of propane hose to go to the generator on my trailer.

   d. My brain will auto lock on some link, which often has nothing to do with the conversation at hand. I am now lost in the wrong place which leads to simple conversations that go on way too long. This causes much stress for others as they can join me on my little wheel of frustration. Hence, loneliness is never a problem.

2. Feeling stupid and inadequate is frustrating.

3. Frustration makes me angry, often VERY ANGRY!

4. Being Very Angry has ugly and unintended consequences.

   a. I become painfully verbal as I lash out at the source.

   b. The anger takes control, it is like watching a movie, and I am the main character. Sometimes a hero, usually the villain.

   c. I have no inhibitions and will get in your face about it.

   d. While I have yet to hurt a human being, many a wall or table will be going to counseling on my dime for the foreseeable future.

5. Being Very Angry, leads to feeling stupid and inadequate! Please see step 2.

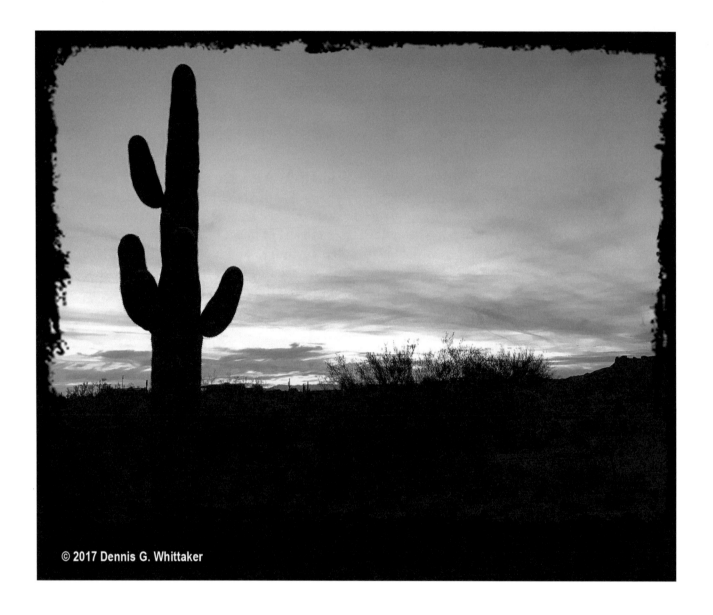

While, agreeably, I would say this single little artifact is enough for any mere mortal to deal with every day, here are a few more, just to keep life interesting:

1. I am a very clean person. I have my wife to blame for this problem, as I often forget to brush my teeth or to take a shower. Therefore, any issues you have with the scent of my deodorant or the need to wear sunglasses when I smile, should be brought to her attention immediately.

2. Redundancy is no longer boring to me.

   a. I have always been a person that could watch a favorite movie or listen to a favorite song many, many times. The difference now being that I go through this process as if it is a brand-new experience.

   b. Example: I have listened to the same SIXX AM album every day for about 6 months now, cause I kinda remember there is an important song that I should focus on. As Hado (the 120-pound Leonberger, pronounced "lean-on-burger") and I take our daily walks, I usually listen to this album. The song "Maybe It's Time to Heal" plays for the 181st time (yup, used my calculator to multiply 6 months times 30 days, plus added an extra day for July), and looked up the name of the song on my music list, to be reminded, seemingly for the first time, that I need to focus on healing and not just being hurt. Sounds like a pretty good plan, I will try to remember that tomorrow.

3. Please don't ask me to "make a decision!"

    a. One thing I remember for some reason, is that I don't make decisions quickly, easily or very well for the most part.

    b. When dining out, to make life easier, more affordable and healthier, I usually tell my wife to order what she wants, and I will eat my share. She knows to not order fish, as no one needs to be reminded about the mess that had to be cleaned up the last time.

    c. If I could make a wish for the one thing that I wish I could remember, it would be this: "Don't be a navigator when driving, EVER!" Let's just say that most of the times that I have watched my life flash before my eyes, have been post cancer, and when I was stupid enough to help. (Help spelled "Shut UP before you kill us all!")

    d. This brings us to making quick decisions, which of course loops us back to the story told in #1 above about Multi-Tasking

4. I like Rice, I have always liked Rice! (Loosely quoting George Orwell's "1984", something about east being at war with the west, or was it the other way around? Thanks George:)! Here is a short list of "Rice-Like" foods that I now enjoy regularly:

    i.   Bell Peppers – any color

    ii. Rice (Other than the Chinese Fried Rice, which is actually only 10% rice, 3% egg, 2% "other" and 40% soy sauce with extra sodium leaving the remainder for the oil used to hold this all together (yumtastic)

    iii. Salads with "so called" (you know who you are, romaine, red leaf whatever, etc.) lettuce

And here is the short list of things I still can't stand:

    i. Broccoli (and broccoli beef, blah blah blah, etc. etc.)

    j. Fish (as noted above)

    k. Cauliflower

    l. Liver

Game animals, especially barbecued

Pre-Cancer I was a total snob when it came to food.

I turned my nose up to an entire food group, something they called "Veggies?" Well, not all of them, but a lot of 'em.

No broccoli, radishes, bell peppers, cauliflower, okra, fish* of any kind, raw carrots and spinach. Pre-Cancer I was a total snob when it came to food.

*While I am fully aware that swimming mammals, such as dolphins and whales are known to have a useful brain, I am not aware of this applying to any fish. Therefore, I am more than comfortable tossing them all in with the so called "Veggies."

Overly nutritious breads, etc.

I always wanted to know what was for dinner so I could audit it and resolve any such concerns by bringing home Pizza because: "I love you soooo much honey, and I don't want you to have to cook"

Food Preferences — After . . .

We eat very healthy these days.

My wife, as it turns out, is a very skilled scientist in the art of cooking. Due to the combination of my listed food phobias, my AHB and my stature in the "workaholics anonymous" group,

I really never gave it the attention it deserved.

She makes homemade breads, yogurt, sauces, etc. etc..

This is my current list of food that I still refuse to eat, under any known circumstances:

Most of which are Veggies:	Some of which are Non – Veggies:
Cauliflower	Organ meat of any kind
Kale	Game Animals
Fish*	
Lima Beans	

Chapter 12

Life After Cancer — How Sweet It Is

"Whip It" by Devo

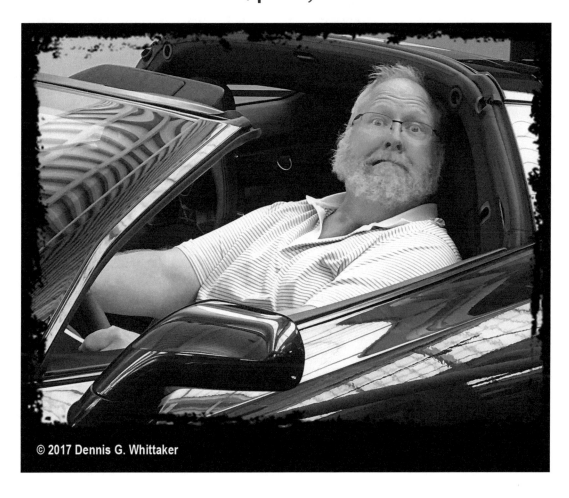

© 2017 Dennis G. Whittaker

I still get up between 2 and 4 every morning, but only to allow mother nature to express herself with the lovely sounds of, well, you get the point. This time of day is no longer the time to get up, get showered and dressed, and head to the home office to start my long day of productivity. No No No, not anymore. I go straight back to bed to saw off a few hundred more z's before it is time to make the morning coffee around 8:30, or 9:16, or? Ahh, who cares, the only important part of this story is this: "I will start working when my coffee does!"

To properly describe my concept of "working" in this new life, it is best stated this way: "I love work,,, I can watch it all day!" (See Dennis'isms for more.) In other words, if you need something done today, put it on a list, remind me once, twice or 22 times, then follow up behind me to make sure you got the result you thought you had asked for. GOOD LUCK!

So, with no real work to be done (see the vicious circle above),, the real work each day is to live a simple, relaxed and stress free life style. Sounds easy, I am sure, but it is quite the exercise for the ol' workaholic over here. The over-reaching and life-long ambition to contribute is a wild horse of sorts and breaking its spirit has been gut wrenching at times. The old mare still wants to rear its ugly head from time to time, and it is painful to whip her back where she belongs.

However, when the old mare remains skulking in its stall (spelled "CELL!" and AKA "EGO") and I simply focus on the day to day. Life is very sweet indeed!

In my world of "I love work,,,, I can watch it all day!," few things satisfy this new work ethic quite like a factory tour. This is the point where this little slogan has the chance to dance with another one, called "Do Whatcha Love and Get Paid for It", which for most of my life has been owning, managing, or touring manufacturing facilities. These days, I earn a living as a disabled person, so I now get paid to research the various factory's where we are, find out about available tours, and go see what they do.

This process, as simple as it sounds, has been a real project for me. After all, there are many steps that need to be followed:

- ❖ Which factories offer a tour?
  - ◆ Please note that the factory that makes "Circus Peanuts" is not open to the public. Trust me on this, so you don't have to go through the FM moment that occurs when you show up and it's closed up like Fort Knox. Not even a basket of free samples outside to pick from.

- ❖ Where are these factories?
  - ◆ While it may be worth driving 6 hours round trip for me to see the Cirrus Airplane Factory, it may not be worth it to my wife, who has to do all of the driving. Trust me on this, so try to avoid hearing and seeing how you often look, when my wife has her own FM moment!

- ❖ What hours are they open?
  - ◆ Showing up for a tour that doesn't run after 1:00 pm at 2:00 pm provides yet another opportunity to feel stupid and inadequate. This is one of the few rules of planning that I have yet to experience, which is a shame, as the FM moments can be so colorful and fun?

❖ Do they require special clothes, like closed toed shoes, etc.
  ◆ Showing up after a 2-hour drive to tour the paper mill in Minnesota is a huge FM moment when you arrive in your new suit, which is shorts, t-shirt and sandals. They require closed toed shoes and recommend a local thrift store to find them. Being on a tight budget, we decide to go back another day/week when we can make a small detour to find this place, with appropriate shoes. Yeah??

❖ What time of year are they available?
  ◆ Continuing on the note right above this one, showing up the next week to learn that the last tour of the season was last week, combined with the pent-up excitement of seeing a tree painstakingly reduced to a piece of copy paper (how humiliating this must be for said tree,) only to find out that you have to wait 5 months, 29 hours and 54 seconds for the next tour, all adds up to one of the most historic FM moments to date.

❖ What days of the week are they open?
  ◆ As a reminder, we sold everything, so we could save money AND travel at the same time. This is called RV-ing! As we painfully make our way through IOWA (Pronounced "No Cell Phone or Data Signals Available for the Next 281 Miles!") we learn the Winnebago Factory is only 30 miles out of the way, my wife says, "No Way!", which I reply to with a simple "Way!" (Thanks Bill and Ted!)

    We happily drive the 30 miles, talking about how cool it will be to see the factory where the RV lifestyle became a reality. We get there, and we are blessed to see that they offer free electric hook-ups in their parking lot, and we can spend the night ("No Way!, Way! Goes here once again! (Bill and Ted's excellent adventure perhaps?) I purposefully and proudly walk towards the door of this surely amazing place, prepared to light a candle and bow to a 2018 motor home. This is when the worst possible thing happened. Yup, the F'ing door was locked. Factory tours are offered M-F, blah blah, blah F'ING blah!

    This led to exactly 30 miles of the FM duet, as my wife and I sang this now familiar tune to a somber bluesish melody as we moved on once more.

  ◆ You are probably asking at this juncture: Did you actually get into any factories for a tour?
  ◆ On the trip in question I have managed to participate in the following tours, in order of excellence:

◈ *Kohler - Wisconsin*
  ◆ Simply unbelievable how this company has managed to innovate their path through every turn in the human story since they started as a simple forger.

    Simple is only used as a reference to the complexity and harmony they have achieved and what I saw while at three of their four factories on campus. It is awe inspiring to watch how they turn scrap steel into a newly forged tub every 26 seconds. Did I mention that I love work,,,, I can watch it all day? This would be a place I could set up a lounger and enjoy watching their work for days on end!

❖ *Cirrus Aircraft*

- The finished airplanes these folks produce are gorgeous! Most things in the factory are on wheels, which allows them the flexibility to build several versions of their 3 models, all at the same time, each one a masterpiece in its own right, and each one has its very own parachute system to make it an extremely safe vehicle to own and fly. Terrific!

❖ *Carr Valley Cheese Factories - Wisconsin*

- Did I happen to mention that my personal belief is that cheddar cheese curds are the best food on the planet? This place cranks out 6000 pounds of these beauties every day they work. The finished product was amazing!!! This one is here in third place because of my addiction to their product. As I have never owned or been on a Harley Davidson, they came in behind them. This is somewhat skewed, as the actual process involved with engineering, manufacturing and ensuring the quality of a Harley engine is way more fascinating than making cheese.

❖ *Harley Davidson Power Plant – Steel Toe Tour - Wisconsin*

- These folks make 250K Harley Engines each year. Highly customized in many cases. Very clean and very efficient place. Most of the work takes place inside of various cells, which don't allow too much of a view of the actual work being done, but from time to time they put a robot in plain view, which is always a treat to see.

Chapter 13

The Other Final Chapter
(still kinda — I'm Not Dead Yet!)

"Not Dead Yet" *by Spamalot*

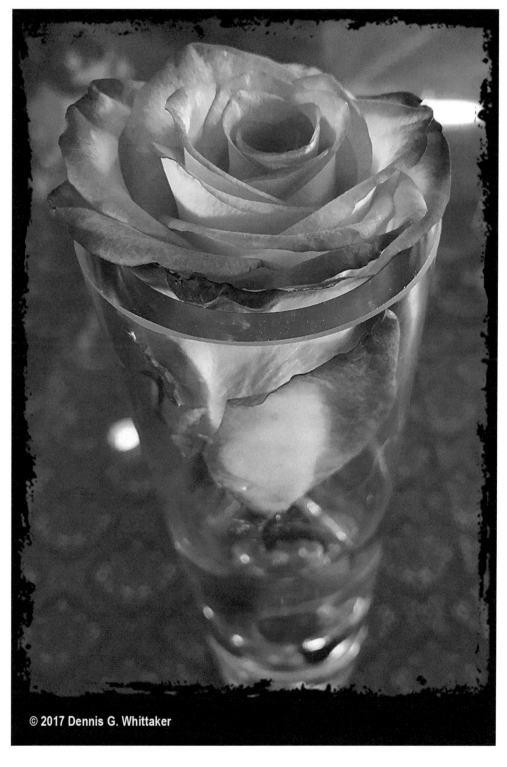

© 2017 Dennis G. Whittaker

Life, is now moving at less than 1 MPH.

The vicious cycle of life before cancer has stopped, at least for me it has.

I am now retired, live comfortably in a 38' travel trailer in a beautiful campground in Columbus, Texas, and will soon be divorced. The artifact of coming clean to some selfish and stupid indiscretions along the way. Things I thought would go with me to the grave. There will always be a very warm place in my heart for the woman that put up with me and all that I was and wasn't for 33 years. Thank you honey.

So, this is where my story takes a funny turn, really. It is the point that I realize that the only way to have the life I crave, is to find a new craving! I know what it is, and I also know that it is true and real. It goes back to the original final chapter, which was all about the quality of a life built on relationships, love and spending time in ways that are truly important. This concept seemed so easy to attain when I started to put this story on paper.

As time moved along however, it turned out there is so much more to adapting to this new better life. The challenges are harder, yet more rewarding. The emotions are stronger, sometimes good, but not always. It turns out that the storm that I survived (cancer) was a class I hurricane and surviving in this new world is the real challenge. It is more of a class IV kind of storm.

I Will Survive! I Will Win! Cancer Be Damned, It Is My Time To Live!

Today, survival is the never-ending process of remembering what is important, or more succinctly, what isn't important. And, as you can see, there is the rub! Remembering isn't really in my portfolio these days. I make a list of the lists that I can't find. On a weekly basis, I have the brand-new realization that I have figured it all out once again.

As I read some of what I have written, and realize, time and again and again, that I have already had this thought, this plan, this realization. Great news! Maybe this time it will stick?

I make a promise to myself, that this time, I will remember to not forget this very important fact. (Yes, the east is at war with the west. The east has always been at war with the west!)

So, for the sake of self-preservation, and to avoid any further mishaps of forgetting what is important, I have made this list of things that aren't important, which should be shorter, easier to remember and easier to find when I need it.

Here is the short list of things that are no longer important in the big scope of things:

- Have a project or two to manage
- Complete something to show the world that I am still worthy!
- Create new, valuable and tangible things to measure my self-worth
- Eat more bacon, chocolate and fresh cheese curds, just 'cause I can
- Work for a paycheck
- Earn a raise or a bonus to represent my contribution
- Drive myself to being better at something than others, at any cost

- Own a bunch of stuff that I can't take with me anyway
- Spend $76 to see the Elvis Graceland, when 20 minutes on Google will do.
- Or **<u>Be somewhere other than right here, right now!</u>**

I am retired at 57. My days are slow and relaxing. I manage my life to be as stress free as possible, which I encourage everyone to embrace sooner than later.

I have time to fiddle with my plastic trombone, listen to music, enjoy my friends and family and find the satisfaction in the very simplest bits and pieces of the human experience.

So, is Cancer my BFF after all?

Absolutely!

After all, if it doesn't kill ya, it will make you stronger and happier:)!

Be well and enjoy the simple things!

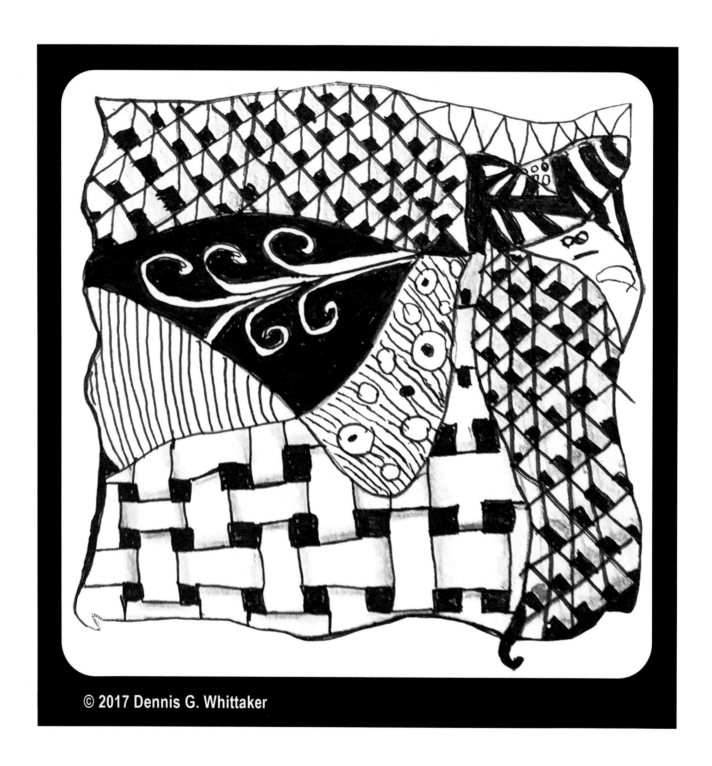

Chapter 14

"The Quipet Sampler"

What! You may ask, be a "Quipet?"

A "Quipet" is a writing style of my own invention, so I believe. It is an observational tale that is told in a very specific way.

Here is how one can quill a "Quipet."

Step 1. Pick a notion, kinda like this example:

"Granny may notion up a chocolate chunk cookie, due entirely to the fact that the chocolate chips had a meltdown earlier, and no longer have the stamina to go it alone:)"

Step 2. Separate your brain from itself for a spell, as this is the only way for a Quipet to present itself.

Step 3. Under no circumstances whatsoever should you over think your thoughts.

Step 4. Please make no effort to make any sense, as this will screw up the entire recipe. However, do do your best to happily and smoothly bounce from one thought to the next:)

Step 5. It is critically important to call back a previously forgotten reference to wrap up the story. If this reference is missing you will have a nice story, but not one worthy of such a fine and expensive title as "Quipet":)

Step 6. Finally, add a personal quote which obtusely wraps it all up, kinda like this this:

"Food for thought!!!!"

Please enjoy roughly 4% of the current "Quipeteria.)!"

Are you a "Factory Second?" 180212

For anyone that feels somewhat out of place, for any reason, today is February 12th, 2018.

Most folks, by the age of 12 months, start to become consumers.

I know this, as this is about the time a child will be reaching for various items at the store.

Let me know if this phrase is familiar to you: "Prnsjzn sbxgc isnavd shrbeb!!," Which can be loosely interpreted as "Not that one, the blue one,,,,,you moron!!"

This, often times, is when the unit's owners, often referred to as "parents or guardians", start to assign titles, or maybe the medical community will assign them.

For this conversation, I will relate all this to traditional manufacturing.

The Quality Department will quickly identify any product anomaly and title it with a "Big Ass Name" (BAN for short.)

This BAN will be reduced to a 3 to 5 letter acronym to reduce cost overruns. (Ever buy a self inking rubber stamp with a bunch of text? Holy Moly!!!)

A few examples:

BAN	ACRONYM
Return to Vendor	RTV
Refurbish and Resale - Factory Second	RFFS
Back to the Drawing Board	BTTDB

If the "Quality Engineer" happens to be a medical doctor, say a Psychiatrist or Psychologist for example, they would define (diagnose) a product (patient) with one or more titles, also reduced to an acronym.

Here are a few that may or may not have been used to define me:

BAN	ACRONYM
Obsessive Compulsive Disorder	OCD
Attention Deficit Hyperactive Disorder	ADHD
AssHoleBergers Syndrome	AHB

These particular acronyms describe defects, or quality control issues, that somehow got past INSPECTOR #15.

For clarity, #15 is solely responsible to ensure that all finished products meets or exceeds all agreed upon specifications.

This is validated with a standardized and comprehensive 129 point quality control process.

Upon completion, #15 will mark each passing unit with his stamp of approval.

You know the one. It is a circle with the number 15 inside of it.

Simply stated, If the recall process wasn't so freaking complicated, most of us would have been sent back to the factory to be adjusted, repaired or replaced a long time ago.

Upon receipt at the factory, we would be re-calibrated, reprogrammed and repainted.

Upon completion of another 129 point QC process, #15 would return to us via FEDEX, COD*.

*Return shipping is only provided when the original owner has purchased the Royal Blue Extended Warranty.

Upon your return, your proud owners will once again see #15's stamp of approval, just to the right of the square that states "Factory Second:)!"

"It's A Boy:)!"

This is a photo of Tommy being created.

During chemo treatments I attended a "do your own thing" painting event with two people who are dear to me.

The event supplied the canvas, brushes and the paint.

I didn't have any idea what to paint, so I closed my eyes and randomly floated the pencil on the canvas.

Within a few seconds, it was obvious that Tommy the Tumor was coming to life.

Tommy became an inspiration to me as my path was now defined by befriending my Tumor in the hopes that he would indeed become my best friend forever.

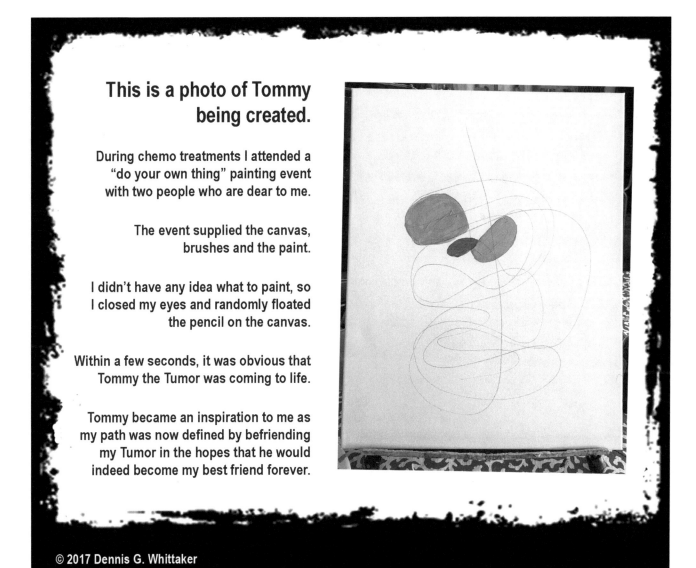

Q2   The Art of "Faux Fishing"

For all those that either don't like fish, or find the process of traditional fishing with bait and a hook somewhat hard to reconcile, today is Thursday, April 25th, 2018.

When I was a kid, Dad, my brother and I would end up on a party fishing boat in San Diego.

I know we had a lot of fun, and while I didn't care to eat the fish, I was more than happy to do my best to land a fish of any size.

We tried fishing in a few Arizona Lakes, and the only thing I caught were tiny sunfish.

Later in Life, Dad and I went on a charter boat in Kauai in hopes of landing a marlin that we could have mounted and hung on our living room wall. I had one on the line, got strapped into the chair, and promptly did exactly the wrong thing as the line snapped. This gave a whole new meaning to the phrase "shoulda seen the one that got away!"

As the kids grew up, we made an effort to share the experience of fishing with them.

Outside of an expensive visit to the trout farm near Sedona, the only thing we ever caught was a nice 7 pound sun burn:)!

Now that I am retired, it would seem that fishing would be a nice pastime, save the fact that it isn't really fair to torture the fish, then not show him the respect of an open flame.

This makes sense to me, so traditional fishing isn't really on my to do list.

It occurs to me, that I could still enjoy the process. A fishing pole, some weights and a bobber is all I need to look and feel the part.

This of course would spawn the interest of other fishers that would stop by, ask if I was having any luck, and potentially deciding that I had found their perfect fishing spot.

My AHB doesn't like that idea so well, so something else occurred to me:)

If I set up 2 or 3 poles and looked real serious about my faux fishing, when folks ask if I am having any luck, I could frown, say no, I have been working this spot for hours, and if I wasn't so lazy I would move on to a better place.

Ahhh, I think I may end up with the catch of the day. A private and quiet spot on the lake, a cold drink and all the time in the world to fish for my next Quipet:)!

"Any Bites????"

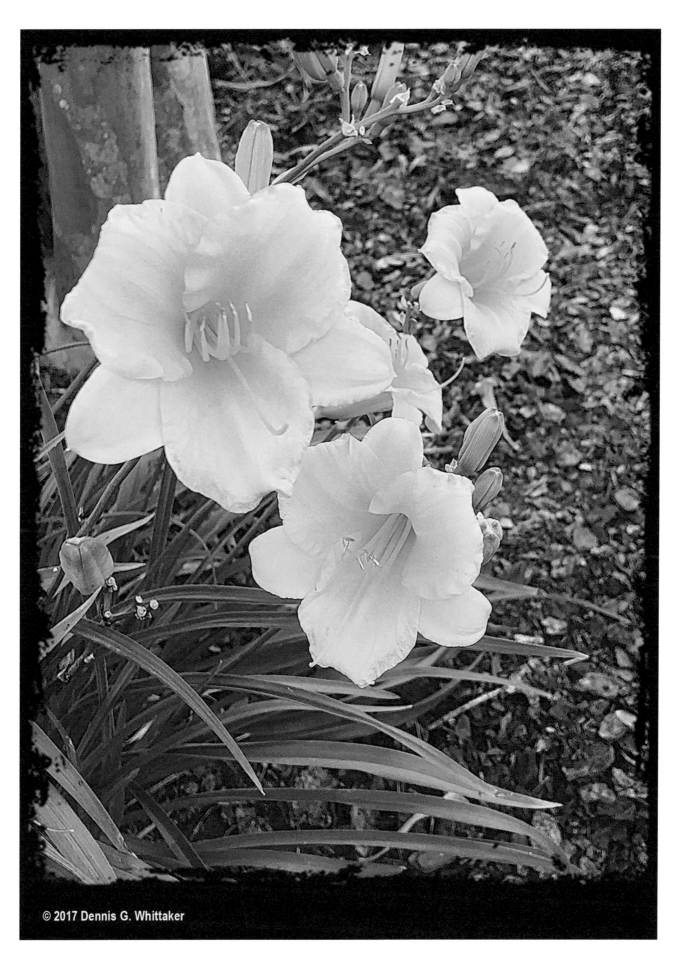

Q3 "Lemon-aide . . ."

For thirsty people everywhere and the makers of any and all refreshing beverages, today is Tuesday, March 23rd, 2018.

This Quipet concept was suggested by a dear friend who prefers cold citrus drinks to coffee at any temperature:)

Every now and again, I come across something that makes no sense to me, whatsoever.

Lemon-Aide is the source of today's confusion.

Being one that is driven to understand how things are made or came to be, topics like this one are fascinating.

I picture the tale unfolding kinda like this:

Man finds an Orange tree, discovers the fruit to be satisfying, at least after it is undressed.

He then finds a grapefruit tree, and while somewhat surprised by the marriage of sweet and sour, adds this new fruit to his diet anyway.

Upon discovering the lemon tree, Man becomes angry, then wildly frustrated.

That's what all men do when they can't make sense of something.

In this case, the dilemma is caused by the similarity to the other items, later grouped and labeled as "Citrus".

It looks similar, albeit smaller and yellower. As with the others, it has been undressed.

The expectation is yet another delicious, possibly tangy item that can be added to the ole diet.

As man's face contorted, twisted and curled, accompanied with free flowing tears, Man invents the very first known use of a 4 letter word.

But that is just simple logic, right?

The dilemma comes in when man figures out somehow, that if this pretty yellow citrus is mixed 20% lemon and 80% high fructose corn syrup, the end result will be sweet, tangy and delicious.

This just doesn't make any sense, AT ALL!!!!

Man is famous for knowing that most things that taste like crap simply don't need to be in our diet (with the exception of Brussels sprouts, fish, seaweed and various forms of birds and wildlife) and we leave 'em alone.

Yet somehow, by intention or accident, lemon-aide, thankfully, was discovered.

This is when it is a nifty that I have already accepted bread into my diet.

Talk about confusing!

Man grows wheat, finds the good stuff, grinds it, leaves it on the counter where mold (yeast) falls in, water is spilled, time passes, someone decides to heat it up, and BAM! we now have bread:)!

If ya can make sense of bread, lemonade is simply a no-brainer:)!

"Fresh Lemon-Aide,,, two bits!"

Q4   Man's Best Friend

For all of our canine pals, today is Sunday, April 22nd, 2018.

Today is a big day for our canine friend, Hado, as he got his rabies booster:)

Hado is a Leonberger. The breed was recognized by the AKC in 2010 and is currently ranked 92 out of 190. I assume this is a simple math error, 'cause they are #1 in my book:)!

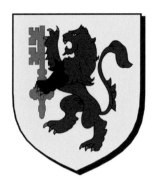

The Leonberger was bred in the 1800's as a gift to the mayor of Leonberg, Germany. The town crest, surprisingly, has a lion(ish) in its crest.

The task at hand was to end up with a new breed, that when trimmed a certain way, will look like a lion.

For the curious, to create the original Leonberger, someone scheduled a menajahtwa with a Saint Bernard, Newfoundland and a Great Pyrenees.

(In other words, I haven't a clue how they made this come to be:))

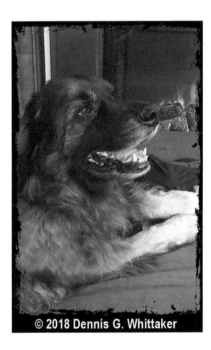

© 2018 Dennis G. Whittaker

Hado has proven to be a wonderful and loyal companion. However, he offers little value as a security dog, beyond his giant 120 pound self.

However, he does come in handy when:

    Ya need a foot rest

    Ya need a foot warmer

    Ya need a conversation piece

    Ya need more exercise

    Ya need an excuse (me so sorry,

       I gotta take care of Hado)

    Ya need a new friend

Hado, which is a Japanese word that means "good energy" has certainly earned his name and his place in my family.

He will bark his baritone bark only when he really wants to come inside, will whine anytime he thinks a treat of any kind may be available, and from time to time will do a little victory dance after he does his business.

Prior to cancer, Hado was more of a possession to me then a companion, but I now consider him to be this man's best friend:)

"Woof Woof,,,,"

Chapter 15

The "After Chapters"

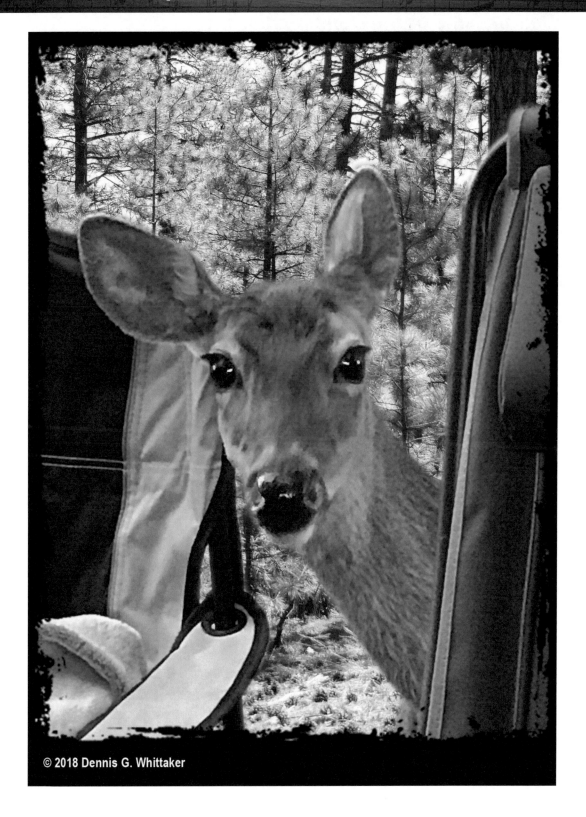

© 2018 Dennis G. Whittaker

I have referenced my legacy a time or two in this book. While I am not claiming to be the first one to ever use any of these, although, I am confident there are at least a couple, I do hereby swear and certify that those that know me, will recognize some or all of these little Dennis'isms.

D1   Dennis-Isms or the Dennis-Ictionary

❖ *I Feel Like a Jackrabbit Fucking a Football.*

- ◆ Source: Ernest Elmer Whittaker, AKA – my dad

- ◆ First awareness of use: When cramming the little Ford Maverick my dad bought with the sole intention of showing me how to rebuild the engine, full of 4 oversized humans. The friend behind my dad, who was driving, was rather tall, as we all were. As Dad moved his seat forward to make room, thereby crushing his body like a slinky into the dashboard, he loudly stated the words "I feel like a jackrabbit fucking a football"

- ◆ Legacy: This has been "the" go to statement for decades between myself and my high school friend. Dozens of people don't need to hear about the origin ever again.

❖ *Damned Gravity! Can't live with it, can't live without it.*

- ◆ Source: Sir Isaac Newton[3], publisher of Philosophae Naturalis Principia Mathematica

- ◆ First Awareness of use: When selling our Kettle Corn, it was only a matter of time with any given customer that a few kernels or an entire bag of popcorn made its way to the ground.

- ◆ Legacy: I am now pretty much incapable of having anything that unintentionally hits the ground to be blamed on, you guessed it,,, Gravity!

❖ *Gotta Breathe, May as Well Enjoy It!*

- ◆ Source: I think this may be one of my own. Doesn't mean that nobody said it before me, I just have never heard it.

- ◆ First Awareness of Use: Can't remember, please read the book for clarification of this defense.

- ◆ Legacy: as most folks at my age of 56, there have been plenty of times to console a friend, employee, family member, spouse, neighbor, etc. As suicide is rarely the path any of these folks are on as they state their frustrations with their job, spouse, economy (personal or national,) health, kids, politics, et al,: At some point over the years,
I came up with the way to finalize any such coaching / fathering/ lecturing moment, with a cheery "Gotta Breathe! May as well enjoy it!"

---

3. "Sir Isaac Newton." sciencekids.com. Science Kids, 2017

❖ *I Would Like a Half-Off Coupon and the Winning Lottery Numbers for Tonight's Drawing.*

- ◆ Source – I doubt if this is an original either but,,,,

- ◆ First Awareness of Use: Probably sometime in 1987ish. At that time, when a server asked if they could do anything else, the answer was usually "I could use a half off coupon, a babysitter for the evening, and the winning lotto numbers. Can you take care of this for me?

- ◆ Legacy: We live in a world of social chit chat. It never ends, and we are all supposed to participate. The comments "how ya doin?" "what's happening?" and every now and again a "Whas UP?" are used as a way to acknowledge that you see another human form, and you are duty bound to acknowledge them in some fashion. The other form, now properly acknowledged, is expected to reply with a standard reply, such as "Good, and You?," "nothing much!" and every now and again, "everythin' man!"

  - ★ My findings have been that folks are taken aback when they serve up one of these social graces, when you return the serve with some actual conversation, like "since you asked,,,,,,,." It takes some practice to pull this off effectively, as they are so accustomed to the canned socially acceptable answers of "Nope, can't think of a thing, everything was great," or "if I eat one more bite I will _____ _____."

❖ *42 is the Answer.*

- ◆ Long story, if you like Douglas Adams, 'nuff said.

❖ *Your Tattoos are Way Cooler Than the Ones I Don't Have!*

- ◆ Source – This one's mine.

- ◆ First awareness of use:

  - ★ At an Army Fort – Selling kettle corn to our dedicated service members

- ◆ Legacy

  - ★ Being 56 in 2017 means that I grew up through a period when folks seemed to come into their own. As this isn't a history book, I will leave it at that. Let's just say that the visibility of tattoos, once only acceptable (well, maybe expected) when covered, or on a soldier or biker. They are now the soul of many personal expressions, and are proudly displayed along with other self-expressions along with hair, clothing, etc.

    This does not in any way interfere with my ability to enjoy the artistic expressions that folks have permanently affixed to their skin. Like any other form of expression, I don't need to understand them, or even like them, to respect them. I can listen to an opera or popular song that is in a language that is completely foreign to me (pun very much intended) and still enjoy the use of the human voice as one of the best instruments anywhere. With all that said: I personally, do not have any tattoos, as my constant fear of needles and distaste for pain in general, exclude me from entertaining such an idea.

However, I am willing to part with my personal business plan that is based on the human desire to take a gamble now and again, literally.

It goes like this:

Go get yourself a giant tattoo of Buddha on your belly and buy yourself a nice collection plate for your "donations." Then you can set yourself up in front of pretty much any casino, race track or convenience store that sells lotto tickets. Folks would rub your belly for good luck, and toss a few bills into your collection plate, otherwise, all that belly rubbing will surely go to waste. This business plan was cleverly designed to allow you to express yourself, write off the expenses for the tattoo & the Tylenol 3 needed to recover, along with all the travel expenses as you would surely be on your way to spread your good fortune with gamblers worldwide!

❖ *"We Used to Have Tile, Now We Have Carpet."*

- ◆ Source – This one's mine.
- ◆ First Awareness of use: Our tiny little dog, which is a 120-pound Leonberger, has 3 full time jobs as follows:
  - ★ Eat, Drink and Beg
  - ★ Sleep (most of the time)
  - ★ Shed (all the time)
- ◆ Legacy: It is practically impossible to take a dog like Hado for a walk without someone asking one of these questions:
  - ▪ He sure must eat a lot (not much really, he sleeps too much to burn any actual calories)
  - ▪ Is he a cross between a German Shepherd and a bear of some kind?
  - ▪ Does he shed a lot?
    - ★ This is where the Dennis-ism:
      "We used to have tile, now we have carpet!" comes from.

❖ *"Problems Don't Go Away, They Just Change."*

- ◆ Source – Unknown – But I have used this one for decades
- ◆ First Awareness of Use – Had to be in the early 1980's-ish
- ◆ Legacy: We go through our daily lives, often wondering what the purpose of all this really is. We're constantly looking to find evidence that we have been successful at, well, pretty much anything. The psychologists in the room would often point out that as humanoids, we will sub-consciously fail at something, as it brings the feeling of success when explained as "I knew that wasn't gonna work!"
- ◆ What brings this "ism" into screaming focus at this moment, which for the historians, is Oct. 27th, 2017, or 3 days or so after being notified of the long-anticipated acceptance for long term disability, my wife and I have found that we still have a few challenges.

Leonberger

A Leonberger is an absolutely gorgeous canine.

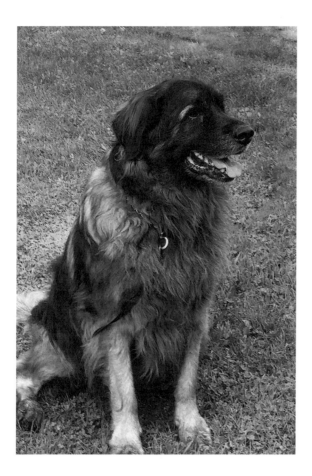

They are known as "The Gentle Giants"

Our Leonberger (HADO) is now 8 years old. We often refer to him as a Lean-On-Berger, cause if you say hi and rub his head he will lean on you with affection.

Roughly one in 239 people recognize him as a Leonberger. Everyone else guesses what he is. We have heard just about every breed with the exception of dachshunds, toy poodles or Shih Tzu

This leads to us telling this story – which is new to most everyone:

Leonberger's were originally bred in the 1800's as a gift to the mayor of "Leonberg, Germany." The town crest is of a Leo (Lion) so they went about the process of engineering the looks of this breed through some mathematical formula that is simply mind boggling to comprehend. It included some percentage of Great Pyrenees, Newfoundland and the Saint Bernard.

For example, I still can't navigate worth a darn, can't make a quick decision about important things like "Do You Want Fries with That?" or to remember to not kiss the woman of your life while chewing gum, especially if for some reason, your lips are covered with some of that nasty "No Sugar Added" chemical of some kind.

So, while the biggest problem we have faced since the day of the cancer diagnosis has been solved, do we get to celebrate this load off our shoulders?

Of course we are, and will continue to do so, but it can be so inconvenient (Pronounced "FM!") at this time to recognize that we still have other things going on that keep our life,,, well,,, human.

❖ *"This is the Best Pizza I Have Had All Day!"*

- ◆ Source – I believe this to be one of mine

- ◆ First Awareness of Use – May 7th, 1991 +-14 years or so?

- ◆ Legacy – I think this is one of my AHB things. As you can tell in my writing, I don't want anybody to call me a liar, question my facts, or just tell me they disagree with me. To avoid these scenarios at all costs, I have literally become a walking and talking disclaimer machine. I really don't know how to turn off this part of my personality, and for good or bad, cancer didn't mess with it, AT ALL!

  So, with that little disclaimer properly noted, I refuse to make a statement like "This is the Best Pizza I have Ever HAD! or that "This is the best sunset ever!" I think these statements are just a lawsuit waiting to happen. How on earth do you go about proving the truth of such a statement? If ya can't back it up, you shouldn't say it.

  However, my AHB has given me permission to state something that has a 99% chance of actually being true, like "this is the best Lunch I have had all day!" or "This Is the Worst Traffic I have Had to deal with ALL DAY!" Go ahead, I dare you, just try to prove me wrong!

❖ *"I Was Wrong One Other Time, So It Is Possible That I am Wrong About This"*

- ◆ Source: mmm, it sounds like one of mine, but I think most of us feel this way but are afraid to actually say it. (As it can't be proven, see Pizza -ism above)

- ◆ Awareness of First Use: January 32st, 2017 plus or minus-ish

- ◆ Legacy: I am an Aries – April 3rd, 1961 for anyone that wants to run my chart, as is my wife, March 22nd, 1955. The sign of the RAM, which usually means that I am strong willed, want to get my own way, and at least for this Aries, like to think that I AM ALWAYS RIGHT! (As in never left!)

  Therefore, when I must concede a point (seems like such a waste of time though, isn't it?) I find it best to protect my well-fed ego from any potential and unnecessary damage over something that is so finite in the whole scheme of things. The statement, "I was Wrong One Other Time, So It Is Possible I am Wrong About This" provides a bit of an out, or a scapegoat, which we all know is the protector of all ego related situations.

  This, at least in the mind and ego of the writer, works to minimize the potential damage (and related medical expenses for the ER, CPR, ICU, and that new leather

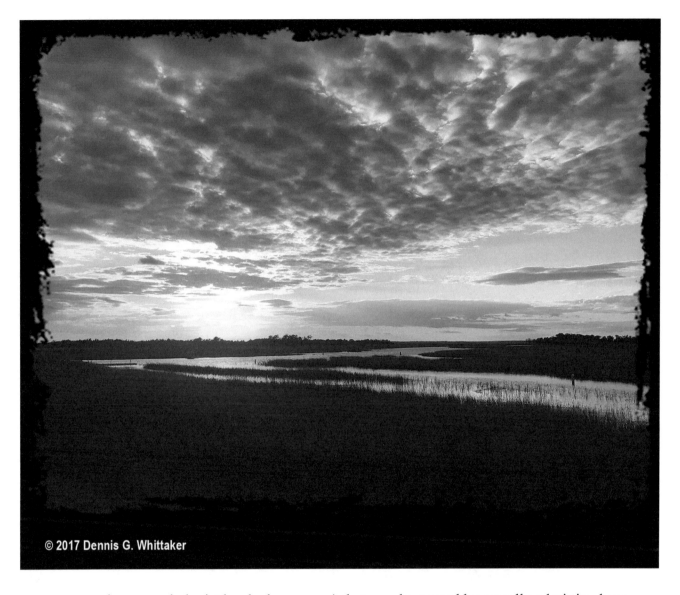

couch my psychologist has had an eye on) that may be caused by actually admitting how many times this horrifying acquiescence may have happened previously

❖ *"No Need"*

- ◆ Source: Heck if I know!
- ◆ Awareness of First Use: Some date greater than 3/1/2016
- ◆ Legacy: As this cancer survivor struggles to accept his new fate as a less productive, potentially more accident prone and mistake prone human form, it has become clear that an easy escape needs to be very handy indeed.
  By looking at any particular task or project, it is much simpler (Pronounced "Your Blood Pressure is 120 over 82. Great Job Dennis!) to simply and flippantly state "No Need!" This simultaneously makes the project unimportant (the project can pay for its own therapy, thank you very much!) and as such, relieves one of any and all responsibility for further action of any kind, including making a note of said project for future consideration.

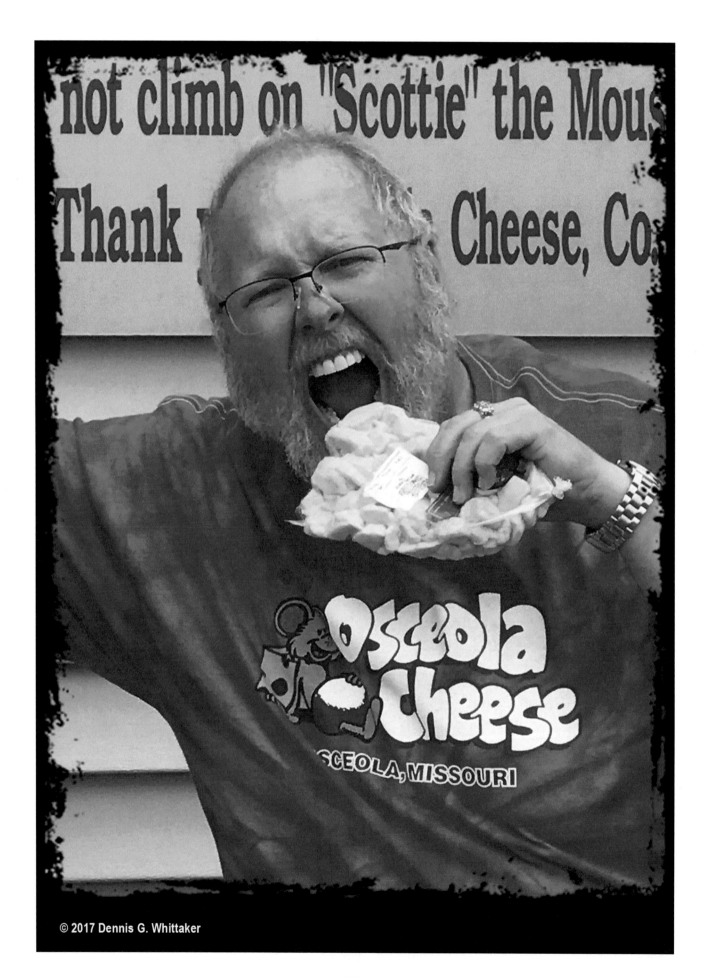

❖ *"I Thought I Had Asked for Extra Cheese?"*

- ◆ Source: Once more the Dennis Person!

- ◆ Awareness of First Use: Since the first time I ordered a pizza with extra cheese and had to send it back with little frown stickers in all the open areas (If ya can see the red sauce, it isn't extra cheese, right?) to make it easy for the pizza chef to know his shortcomings, remake pizza to appropriate specifications, ask the pizza god and the cheese god for forgiveness, and try, if at all possible, to carry on making yet another pizza pie.

- ◆ Legacy: This is one of those that I create a never-ending list of times I had to state "I thought I asked for Extra Cheese? Or some version thereof. For this tale, I will keep it to two simple stories.

  - ★ This one time, at band camp (movie chuckle intended), I ordered this pizza with "As Much Cheese as It Can Possibly Hold!" I realize this isn't a scientific measurement, due to the type and style of crust, the ambient temperature and the moisture content of the cheese(s.) However, I think it is safe assumption that the weight of the cheese would cause the crust some level of anxiety when picked up, and if the cheese comes from a good family, would create one of those unmanageable strings that we chase around with our arms and mouth as we try desperately to cut it from its source. Needless to say, this particular pizza had no signs of trouble and was ridiculously easy to separate each slice. May it hang its head in shame!

❖ This other time, not at band camp, I went to one of my favorite pizza places. What, you might ask, would make me call any pizza restaurant a favorite? Clearly, they have proven themselves, time and again, of being willing and able to apply the appropriate amount of cheese to any pizza ordered with, you guessed it, "Extra Cheese!" So, you can imagine the feelings of shock and betrayal when such a fine establishment, which must now be under new management by some stupid cheese-miser, delivers "the usual" and it doesn't have even a fraction of the appropriate crust bending amount of cheese on top. I asked my waitress this simple question: "I had asked for extra cheese. I even stated that you could not possibly put too much cheese on this pizza for my liking, did I not?" She made some ugly noise about how she had put it on the ticket, it's not her fault, it's the pizza chefs fault, and blah blah F-ing blah.

In hopes of avoiding and removing any possible question about my request for extra cheese, I kindly asked this young lady this: "What exactly, should I ask for when ordering a pizza to ensure that it has plenty of that gooey goodness on top?" She contemplates the question, so I knew she was empathetic to my concern, and wanted to provide a useful answer: "Maybe, you should ask for a MOUNTAIN OF CHEESE!" I thought this over for a few seconds, and asked a simple follow up question: "So, if I order a pizza here, with a MOUNTAIN OF CHEESE, I will be a happy guy?" She shrugged her shoulders and then stated, "I doubt it" then happily went back to her routine.

❖ *"Averages"*

- ◆ Source: I can't claim any authorship to this mathematical term, and don't believe it's first use is of value to this story.

- ◆ Awareness of First Use: Likely in grade school.

- ◆ Legacy: I have found that averages are a very clever invention indeed. Anyone who has seen their car or home owner's insurance skyrocket over a simple claim can appreciate my point of view on this topic. There are 10's of millions of drivers in the US, and a handful of us end up in an accident from time to time. The 10K or even an entire $1M of expenses from an accident would ultimately cost the average driver a few pennies a year. Correct me if I am wrong, but I believe that is exactly the reason we all run out to buy insurance in the first place. If something goes sideways in life, the entire community of friends, neighbors and the like will happily jump in to help.

  Why will they help? I think I already answered this one.

  The insurance company, which often markets themselves under slogans involving big hands or good neighbors immediately begin charging higher premiums to the victim of the accident or issue. They do this to you even though you were not at fault when someone else slammed into your car at a stop light.

- ◆ Another vicious circle starts with this conversation:

  - ★ Insured person: "Why did my rates go up?
  - ★ Insurance company: "Because you were in an accident!"
  - ★ Insured person: "But it wasn't my fault. This shouldn't affect my rates, right?
  - ★ Insurance company: "It doesn't work that way"
  - ★ Insured Person: "Why not"
  - ★ Insurance Company: "I don't know really, it is what the computer says.
  - ★ Insured Person "So you now have two people paying the costs for the same accident, how convenient!"
  - ★ Insurance Company "By the way, our office will be closed next week!"
  - ★ Insured Person: "Must be nice! Why's That?"
  - ★ Insurance company: "We had a really great quarter, so the neighbors with big hands are taking everyone in the office on a cruise to the Bahamas!"
  - ★ Insured Person: "FM!!!!!!!

❖ *"All I Need,,,,"*

- ◆ Source: I have to give credit to the movie "The Jerk" with Steve Martin and Bernadette Peters. As they went from rags to riches to rags, Steve runs around half dressed grabbing up a lamp and a chair and a few other things, while stating, loosely quoted as "All I need is this lamp, and this chair, and this other thing"

- Awareness of First Use: Roughly 15 minutes after seeing the movie a second time.
- Legacy: This statement has become a go-to comment with my wife and I. It works in just about any setting, any time of day, and will go with both your summer and autumn wardrobes. Wine Pairing suggestion: This will go well with both Dasani or Aquafina!

❖ *"Shosh"*

- Source: My daughter
- Awareness of First Use: Roughly 2/3 of a full moon that occurred after a full moon, but not before one of those sliver moons that for some reason, simply can't be trusted.
- Legacy: My daughter had hearing problems that were later cleared up with some tubes in her ears. Until that time, she was a tad behind with her language. Hence, words like "Shower" were lovingly turned into non-words, like "Shosh!" It took a night or two, but we soon learned that when a naked 3-year-old ran through the house towards the little room with a shower in it gleefully yelling "Shosh!," it was time for said child to take a shower.

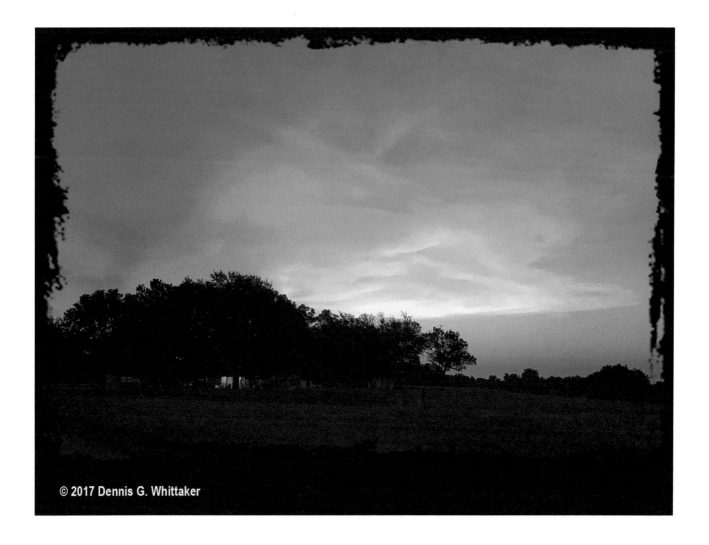

❖ *"There Must Be 51 Tits Up There!"*

- ◆ Source: Ernest Elmer Whittaker, aka my Dad

- ◆ Awareness of First Use: I could probably write a book with the only subject being my dad, who always had a way of doing and saying things that were educational and heartwarming at the same time.

- ◆ Legacy: When I was 18, my dad fulfilled his fatherly duties by taking me to a Las Vegas show, which at the time, being 1979, ensured that at least some percentage of the staff had signed paperwork that stated they were to purposefully leave any clothing that would normally be worn between the person's waist and neck would be left in the dressing room. More often than not, the folks that signed these contracts were females. They didn't have to be the prettiest girl in the room, as that role was saved for the gal that got to wear all her clothes and could sing or dance better than any of the other girls. This 18-year-old didn't have the ability to focus on important things like cheekbones or perfect teeth, 'cause on the stage at the time the pretty girl was singing and dancing her heart out, there were 51 tits on the stage, happily bouncing and swaying to the music.

  Each of the 51 tits was performing a special dance, seemingly just for me.

  I unconsciously decided it would be simply rude to not give this performance 110% of my attention, so was therefore unable to count to two, let alone 51. Luckily for me, my dad, having experienced this marvel previously, was kind enough to do the math and to let me know that yes, there must be 51 tits up there!

❖ *"I Tried to Help, But Nothing Happened"*

- ◆ Source: If this isn't one of mine, I should shoot myself.

- ◆ Awareness of First Use: Sometime after the 51 tits had changed my life forever.

- ◆ Legacy: I have always had a desire to help and be productive. This enthusiasm was not always welcomed, as the person that needed the help didn't know it, or at the very least, wouldn't admit that they needed it. From these humble beginnings, I recognized this: "I tried to help, but nothing happened"

  Later in life, I recognized this could also be true when someone either needed or wanted my help, but for some stupid reason, I was actually unable to help. Being one to take a great deal of pride being both smart and helpful, this has proven to be one of the most confusing conundrums ever!

❖ *"Is Your Shirt Battery or Solar Powered?"*

- ◆ Source: This is a Dennis'Ism

- ◆ Awareness of First Use: It was the winter of 2011 at the PX at Fort Carson

- ◆ Legacy: While offering samples of our "Ridiculously Delicious Kettle Corn" to pretty much anything with a pulse that came within 37.28 feet of me, it was only a matter of time before a person came by wearing the latest seasonal color, which of course, was fluorescent anything. The usual orange, changed to yellow, then green. Blue, for all its masculine overtones, never had a chance.

Being one to find something to say to these folks, I came up with this line "Is your Shirt (shorts, leggings, eye shadow, shoes, etc.) Battery or Solar Powered?" Rarely did I get an answer, but I almost always got a chuckle or guffaw for my clever use of the English language.

And while I did my best to find out what powered these insanely bright colored garments, this, as with so many other things, will likely be left in the ever-growing collection of things unanswered.

❖ *"What Did John Want?"*

- ◆ Source: College friend

- ◆ Awareness of First Use: It was an evening, a cool breezy evening in the summer of 1981, or was it 1980, or,,,,???? Well, it was at a Movie Theater in the South-west

- ◆ Legacy: My friend and I, both being of sound mind(ish) and round bodies, were always able to devour more than our share of food, especially foods that were full of everything we aren't supposed to eat, like fats, sugars, nitrates, high fructose corn syrup, red dies 1 through 1M, you get the picture. We had enough experience to somehow know that an appropriate amount of these foods to consume during the course of an average movie was exactly this: One Soda, any size, 1 Serving of popcorn, and 1 single candy bar.

This was a time for us to let the world know that we were not stupid, as we do in fact know that ordering and consuming any more than the socially acceptable amounts stated above, would be frowned up (PRONOUNCED "LOOK AT THOSE TWO PIGS! THEY HAVE ENOUGH JUNK FOOD TO FEED AN ARMY! I NEVER,,,,,,,:!"

This was the day that I learned just how deep and considerate a thinker my friend really was. Just as all the naysayers in line behind us started to say, "LOOK AT,,,,," my friend quickly asked me this one very simple question: "What did John Want?" I didn't know a John at that time, and he certainly wasn't with us. However, we were now able to order 2 more candy bars and a hot dog under this illusion of a disguise.

❖ *"Squish and Pivot"*

- ◆ Source: This is a pure Dennis'ism for sure!

- ◆ Awareness of First Use: When the kids were just starting to feed themselves.

- ◆ Legacy: Our society, while more relaxed than any that came before us, are hung up on what is often referred to as "A Proper Place setting" Earlier civilizations had clearly stated that this would include the following apparel, which was to be "set" at the dining room table.

  2 Forks – One for Salad, which must be between 3/8" and 1" shorter than the other fork.

  2 Knives, one to be used specifically for butter. Due to the unique molecular structure of butter, it was critical that only the finest and properly honed of all knives be trusted in its presence.

  2 Spoons, one for the soup, since most folks are most hungry at the beginning of the

meal, and this huge spoon is the perfect instrument to transfer this boiling bowl of leftovers into our face. The other spoon, often not used at all may be used to somehow twirl certain Italian bread products, called pasta, into a maneuverable shape to transport to one's mouth. Other uses may include desert, but that usually comes out with the appropriate tool at the right time.

2 Plates, one for the salad, which is important, since we already have a special fork just for it, one for the meal, which is just as important for the same stupid reason.

1 Bowl, for said soup.
Many of us today either don't have a dining room, and if we do, we have forgotten it's intended purpose. We all know now that the room with a telly is the appropriate place to dine, so why not put a foosball table in that other room that we never, ever use? In this so called "Dining Room" we set our table by grabbing the exact instruments that will most efficiently transfer the meal into our face. As any utensil that leaves the traditional kitchen / dining area must be washed, dried and placed back in the "Silverware Drawer," it is important to learn how to use the most basic set of these utensils, as we don't want to interfere with our telly time, right? That is why, at the first sign of an ability for the child to shovel their own food into their own faces, I invented, or maybe simply coined the phrase "Squish and Pivot."

Done properly and with an appropriate attitude, it is often possible to eat even the most robust and complete meal with a single fork. However, this isn't as easy as it sounds. Understanding that children learn a foreign language faster than an adult, logic would follow that it would also apply to the many learned tasks of eating.

Using the "Squish and Pivot" technique properly, even a young person can cut through and manage to eat meals that could be only be enjoyed previously with a very sharp and dangerous thing called a "Steak Knife."

So, for one reason or another, be it self-preservation, somehow knowing the kids may tire of me at any time, are better left unarmed, or simple laziness, as I was gonna be the one that would have to clean, dry and store the extra utensils,,,,,,

"Squish and Pivot" to the rescue. Many a minute was spent with each child teaching them to apply an appropriate amount of pressure to cut off the appropriate size piece of dinner, then with the same amount of pressure, to pivot the fork back and forth, until such time the appropriate piece of dinner had been separated from its parental units, and therefore, is ready to eat. I have now properly educated two generations of Whittaker's on this important strategy. I can only hope that these young folks work to preserve this important legacy for all future generations!

❖ *"Car Full of Losers,,,,, "*

- Source: This is a pure Dennis'ism for sure!
- Awareness of First Use: When driving in Apache Junction with our grandson
- Legacy:

From Time to time, we all say exactly what we think, then we get to deal with the fallout. In this case, I looked to the car beside us, which was an older model, lots of putty and red primer. The amount of music can't be measured in decibels, as it is beyond the ability for such measurements. There were many youths in the vehicle, pronounced "Punks" with their special clothes and attitudes. This is when I said exactly this out loud: "Car Full of Losers." My wife and I laughed about this spontaneous moment, then forgot all about it. Our grandson, on the other hand, did not. We know this, because about 2-3 weeks later while driving somewhere else, our grandson announced loudly "Car Full of Losers" which of course caused a chain reaction of these events:

1. Find car to validate if this statement was accurate, which according to my definition above, was completely accurate.

2. Perform a series of breaths in an attempt to avoid supporting these shenanigans by laughing hysterically.

3. Figure out a way to get our grandson to understand, that like all swearing, it is perfectly okay for an adult to use the language, however, god will strike you down if at age 8, or any age below 18, for doing a forbidden thing.

Did I say that out loud just now?

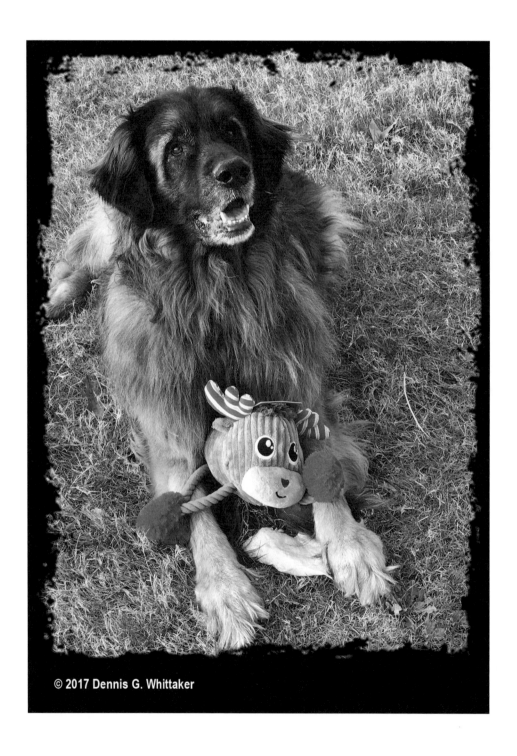

Oldest Kid in School that Still Believed in Santa

While I stated earlier that I wasn't the best dad ever, I wasn't the worse one ever. Or was I??????

It probably didn't help that my brain truly believed that when my kids grew up and ended up a shattered mess and decided to share it with the world on Oprah, Dr. Phil or what's his name that loved to tell the 17th lover that "YOU ARE THE FATHER! I would have a full and complete understanding of what I did exactly to cause this incident to occur!!

A NEW Christmas Story

I don't know what the exact age is that kids are supposed to stop believing in Santa Claus, but I do know that my daughter was the oldest in her "?th" grade class that still believed. Why? I thought you would never ask.v

One Christmas Eve, I decided it would be good to put a little more magic into Christmas Eve, so I made an annual tradition of this fun and classy way to keep the Santa dream alive!

This is what'cha do:

- ◆ Phase #1 – The preparation for the launch!
  - a. Have each kid write a note to Santa Claus
  - b. Fold the note up into a small square, but keep track of how you fold it
  - c. Fold a blank paper (same kind for sure) the same exact way out of sight of the kids,
  - d. Go to the local party store and make a big deal with your kids as they select their favorite color balloon (I think some of you are already catching on??)
  - e. Slip the "fake / blank" note into the balloon and give it to the clerk to fill with helium.
- ◆ Phase #2 – The actual launch
  - a. After you get back home, and at a time the entire family can join in, it is time to launch the Santa Notes into the sky for easy retrieval by Santa
  - b. It is very important to tell the kids exactly this, as the illusion may fade otherwise: "It's is critical that you send Santa his Christmas Eve Note from the same exact home that you are going to wake up in, as the balloon lets him know exactly where to deliver your Christmas Presents, Okay? "(It is important to confirm they understand the importance of this part of the process. If they don't believe that Santa will find the balloon, you can forget all about them having a hard time going to sleep with the anticipation that is soooo important here!)
  - c. Go inside the house and have the kids prepare your favorite snacks to leave out for Santa. It is critical that you like what is left out, because it is just rude not to eat at least some of what your kids were so thoughtful to place perfectly on the Santa Plate, right?
  - d. Have the kids place the food in a safe and conspicuous place so "Santa" can find it

as his reward for messing with your head in such a fantastical fashion as this! (Notes to self: DO NOT EVER ALLOW THE CHILDREN TO SET THE SANTA PLATE ANYWHERE NEAR THE CAT LITTER. PERIOD!!!)

- Phase #3 – The preparation for the Landing

    a. The kids are all tucked in bed after doing such a fine job writing such a sweet note to Santa. (They didn't say "LIKE" even once, like, ya know what I mean?, helped pick out the balloons and launching them, and even taking their time to prepare your snack and putting it in a safe place, and finally going to bed and closing their eyes real tight (Or Santa won't bother coming, or any other idle threat you prefer to use on your defenseless little ones)

    b. Make a stiff drink, then make it a double as a reward for being brilliant enough to remember all this after 1 to 364 days ago when you read it, and actually doing this on the busiest day in the year for most folks, which is actually Christmas Eve. (If water is your idea of a stiff drink, as it is mine, you will need at least a 32-ounce insulated drink cup in order to make a double. These are available for $10 from RTIC or Walmart, or $4754.32 for an original Yetti model)

    c. Take out the original note at this time. If the paper is blank, no offense, but you are a baboon (or dingbat, idiot, moron, dufus, or just plain old or toooo busy to pay attention to such a minor detail) and forgot to switch the notes from the first phase, and this whole exercise has become a huge waste of your time and money. Good luck tomorrow!!!!!!

    d. Take your finest gold fountain pen out of your antique solid oak roll top desk (or Bic pen off your counter) and answer the note to your child, in your own words, as YOU are the only REAL Santa your kids will ever know. This is your perfect chance to manage your kiddy's expectations, right?

Here is an example for you;

"Sorry Izabel, I know you had your heart was set on the new Ken Doll from Apple that is anatomically correct and will answer any question you have about just about anything, in any language and in any accent, but my silly elves didn't buy enough of those nuclear infused battery thingies that make them work. I will do my best to manage them better next year. For this year, please enjoy, with my love and merriest wishes, a brand new, high quality and thoroughly tested, anatomically correct pair of socks and matching t-shirt. I sincerely appreciate how good you have been these past 364 days, but do expect you to do a little better with your math homework this coming year.

Chapter 16

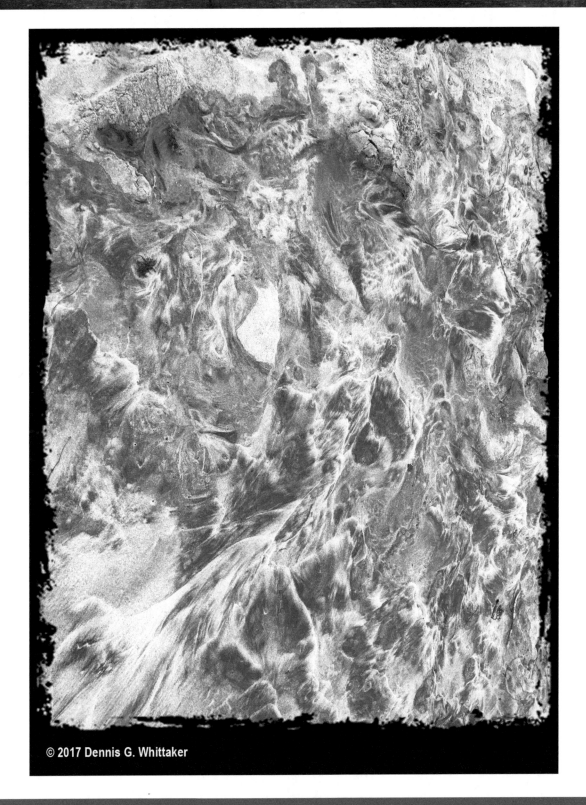

© 2017 Dennis G. Whittaker

What is this, dare you ask?　　　　*See page 105 for answer.*

- Source: My son

- Awareness of First Use: Roughly in the spring, summer, fall or winter sometime in 1990 or 1991

- Legacy: My son, at the age of 2-3 years old was a lot of really cool things, however, he was not a movie buff of any kind. Multiple times (pronounced "Every Single Time!") he would loudly ask, roughly 9-12 minutes into any movie "Is this the over part?"

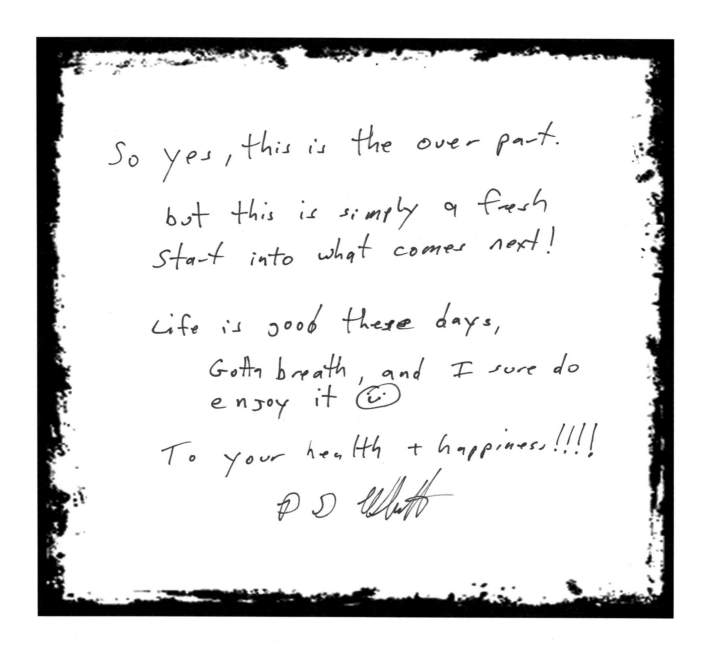

Image References

What is this, dare you ask?   Answer:

This photograph is a close-up shot of sand at a beach in California. It makes for an excellent thought provoking and brain twisting image for family and friends, especially those who are avid photographers themselves.